Advance praise for Susan Carol Stone's
At the Eleventh Hour: Caring for My Dying Mother

"An exquisite exploration of the heart . . . Susan allows us to accompany her on the path that leads through death to birth—for death in the family can move us toward the birth of our own deepest being. A must-read for all who want to aid and support their parents through the dying process."

Ondrea and Stephen Levine
Who Dies? An Investigation of Conscious Living and Conscious Dying

"Susan Carol Stone's memoir is honest, compassionate, and filled with practical wisdom. Her clear and mindful view of living/dying shines through each page."

Dale Borglum
Executive Director, Living/Dying Project

"This poignant remembrance of the passing of a life relates, with loving insight, the personal growth that occurred between daughter and mother during their last days together."

Cheryl Hardy
Director of Communications, Colorado Center for Healing Touch

"*At the Eleventh Hour* offers a heartwarming and inspirational perspective on caretaking for a dying parent. With clarity and sensitivity, it illustrates how communication bridges can be built at any stage of a significant relationship. This book takes us on a spiritual journey that we all share."

Matthew Flickstein
Swallowing the Ganges: A Practical Guide to the Path of Purification
Director, The Forest Way Insight Meditation Center

"In *At the Eleventh Hour,* Susan Carol Stone writes skillfully about the fear and concern, the joy and pain of caring for her dying mother. Weaving the truths of Buddhism with her mistakes and successes as a daughter and caregiver, Susan allows the reader to see the human side of her spiritual practice. A worthy read for anyone interested in untangling romanticism from the subject of death."

Rodney Smith
Lessons from the Dying

At the Eleventh Hour
Caring for My Dying Mother

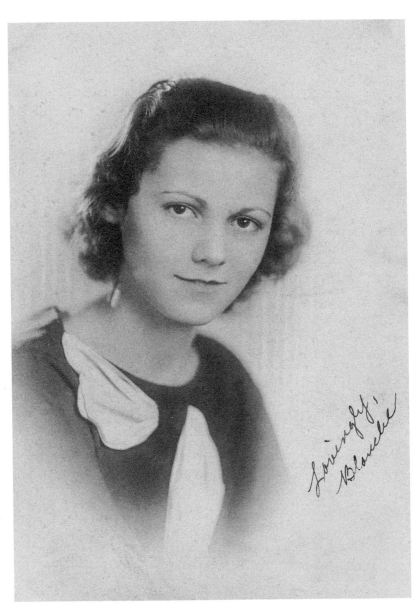

Blanche Olschansky Stone

At the
Eleventh Hour
Caring for My Dying Mother

susan carol stone

 Present Perfect Books

Publisher's Cataloging-in-Publication

Stone, Susan Carol.
    At the eleventh hour : caring for my dying
mother / Susan Carol Stone. -- 1st ed.
    p. cm.
    LCCN: 00111479
    ISBN: 09630784-5-3

    1. Stone, Susan Carol. 2. Stone, Blanche.
3. Mothers and daughters--Case studies. 4. Terminally ill
--Family relationships. 5. Terminally ill--Home care.
6. Bones--Cancer--Patients--Biography. 7. Terminal care
--Religious aspects--Buddhism. I. Title.

HQ759.S76 2001   306.874'3
                    QBI01-200745

Cover and design by the Design Den, Pocatello

Present Perfect Books
P. O. Box 1212, Lake Junaluska, NC 28745

To Blanche Stone—Mom—instead of the book of poetry

And to caregivers—
those who have been and are, with loving respect,
and those who will be, with encouragement

Contents

An Offering

Life happens while we're busy making other plans, as the wise man said, and so does death. Living and dying. They bleed into each other incessantly. In meditation we can discover that we die a little death with each outbreath, begin afresh with the inbreath. And the space between?

In 1996, I was living at Shasta Abbey, a Buddhist monastery in northern California, preparing to become a monk, when my mother was diagnosed with non-Hodgkins lymphoma in the bones, an uncommon form of cancer. I went to St. Louis to live with her for six months as she underwent chemotherapy. Afterwards, I returned to the Abbey, but I was back in St. Louis at the end of the year, just as her condition was diagnosed as terminal. I stayed on until she took her last in-out breath and after.

Friends sometimes commented about my willingness to put my life "on hold." In fact, it wasn't on hold. This living with dying *was* my life, every minute of it. Sometimes it seemed impossibly hard. It was also full of wonder. Not only the nuts and bolts of the matter—not only that events yanked me from my intended path and plunked me down, like Dorothy in Oz, in a place I hadn't planned to live; not only that my mother's and my relationship at that late hour became a garden full of quiet surprises, some of them with thorns—those things were wonderful enough.

But beyond that, a greater wonder: the wonder of discovering the *equivalence of experience*. Living and dying, the pleasant and the unpleasant, what one wants and what one doesn't—I found that on some deep level, they are the same.

Something in us rebels at the notion, finds it appalling. It's hard to accept that an hour of slow dying alone in the midst of a war, for example, or the loss of a son or daughter is no different than a quiet hour shared with loved ones or a ramble along a beach at sunset. Of course they're different! Naturally we prefer happy experiences. Naturally we want to avoid the painful ones. But natural preferences can lead us to doggedly wrap ourselves in them and snuggle there. Something deeper than my rebellion knows that in the doggedness, in the wrapping and the snuggling are problems. And those problems are both subtle and seismic.

When we try to lay aside that blanket and just experience the cold, if it is cold, and the heat, if it is hot, without struggling against it, when we strive to live with awareness and caring, simply doing our best as circumstances require, then these moments become our heart's-offerings to the universe. Then, we begin to know the equivalence of experience, for—whether bright, neutral, or agonizing—all experience can be infused with the same deep joy.

For me in St. Louis, this joy sprang from two sources. First, from the knowledge that, despite my bumbling, I was trying to live, based on moral principles, as the moments instructed. They were teachers, these moments. Like manna in the desert bestowed upon the wandering Hebrews in Biblical times, they sustained me, providing exactly what I needed, though not necessarily what I wanted, to exist perfectly. In their particularity—in the hum of the refrigerator, in the grassy view from the bay window partly blocked by the ivy-covered trunk of a massive mulberry tree, in Mom's feeble "Honey?" from the other room, in a fugitive fear that often ran just beyond my reach, and in the almost tactile yearning for what was absent—in all these things, in each moment, was instruction. When I listened closely enough without getting caught in my own preferences, the moments pointed the way and showed me what needed to be done next. Clarity was right there. All I needed to do was notice.

Second, the joy came from the quiet, refreshing energy released by my meditation. I can't dwell on this, for it can't be conveyed in words. It seems fitting to say, however, that during my stay with my mother, my most intimate companion was my Buddhist training, my abiding practice in finding the clear place. Even when I forgot it, which was often enough, my intention was to remember.

I need to explain something here. Being a Buddhist or training with Buddhist practices does not necessarily carry the same meaning as adherence to a faith in the Judeo-Christian-Muslim tradition. Buddhist practice is based on principles different from those of the formal faiths with which we Westerners are familiar. It is not primarily a belief system or a faith. The Buddha, who was a historical figure, advised a group of listeners some 2,500 years ago not to believe anything he said. He urged them to "come and see for yourself." Check it out, test it. It was the original do-it-yourself approach.

The goal was nothing less than the attainment of inner peace and clarity. The Buddha discovered and, for forty-five years, diligently taught means of training—actually retraining—the mind to open to its own proper birthright, enlightenment. That potential is present in all people, but it is usually obscured because the mind is so lost in opinions, aversions, desires, and confusion.

Buddhist practices are without doctrinal content. There is no need to memorize a credo or to subscribe to a theory. Contemporary Westerners are finding that they needn't even be Buddhist to follow these practices. Regardless of formal religious affiliation, one can practice, for the training doesn't conflict with beliefs, working as it does on a different level. These practices become interiorized and can take one deeper into one's own religious tradition.

I came to Buddhist practice from a background of little formal religious observance, but with a deep sense of spirituality. I am grateful beyond expression to this training and to those who have helped me on my spiritual path. There are many. Especially I want to thank Reverend Gosung Shin in the Washington, D.C., area whose teaching grounded me in Zen Buddhism, and Reverend Master Eko Little, Abbot of Shasta Abbey Buddhist Monastery, where I lived for two years. I'm grateful to Reverend Master Eko especially for his long-distance spiritual counseling during the months my mother was dying as well as afterwards. At a time when elements in my life were blowing around like tumbleweeds in the desert, these conversations helped me hear the steadiness in the wind. More recently, the teaching of Matthew Flickstein opened for me the heart and clarity of Vipassana, or Insight Meditation. I am profoundly grateful to him and to the Venerable Henepola Gunaratana, at whose monastery, the Bhavana Society, I gained training in that tradition.

During the months of my mother's dying, friends occasionally urged me to write about my experiences. The suggestion didn't appeal. Living those experiences was challenging enough. Writing about them seemed more than I could undertake. Then, three or four weeks before Mom died, the suggestion struck with compelling force, as though it were a fresh idea. What really struck me was *how* to write: lightly, with the love and humor that we shared. Not a systematic discourse laden with angst or purporting to provide transcendent wisdom about dying and caregiving, but stories celebrating our experiences together, the poignant as well as the raw and tedious ones. And, too, those that were fun.

For Mom and I did have fun, right in the midst of it all. The finality of the circumstances gave a special savor to what we did. We each tried to allow that savor to be expressed lightly and in laughter, when we found the chance. We became friends across our differences, slowly saying what needed to be said, sharing some, but not all, of our reactions to the traumas of those months. And we each grew internally.

When I told Mom I was thinking of writing about our life together, I asked if she would like me to do it. Already bedbound and scarcely eating or drinking, she smiled, nodded, and whispered, "Yes."

Mom would have written a very different account of these months if she had written at all, which is unlikely, my shy mother who found her voice only among those she'd known long and comfortably. Yet in a real sense, this book is her offering as well as mine. We hope you enjoy it.

And I hope you find encouragement in our stories as you grapple with your own dilemmas. Each relationship and situation is unique, of course. What nourishes one likely won't another, and what is nourishing one moment in a given relationship may be noxious the next. It's a process of continual fumbling. Mom and I decided she'd become a hospice patient and that I'd live with her at her home until the end. We felt our way from there.

And so, if you are tussling with your issues, whether they involve dying, or caring for someone who is, or any of the other issues without number that we face as we live and die, then maybe our stories will be a small support to you. Fumbling loves company, doesn't it?

While this book tells my mother's and my stories, the voice is mine, and as I wrote, I felt as though I were learning to sing. These weren't simply stories; they were songs. Finding my voice was a process of discovery, for I hadn't expressed myself in such a way before. I loved the singing; yet, it demanded much more than I had expected. In early versions, I largely took cover behind events concerning Mom. I wrote as a silent observer, the fly-on-the-wall approach. I soon realized, however, that this made only half-stories, half-songs. It was an evasion. The stories needed to be made whole by the inclusion of my reactions and experiences, even some of those that weren't directly related to Mom, for all were part of life as I cared for her. This led to the disclosure of information about myself that I hadn't been prepared to share.

Among other things, I realized that I couldn't tell the stories without referring to the spiritual training that informed my actions. In this book of stories-songs, I sometimes needed to present Buddhist teachings. To do this, without being didactic, to create a work of celebration and yet one clear to readers unfamiliar with Buddhist spirituality, was a challenging task. Whether I've succeeded or not, I am grateful to you for listening. I bow to you on your path, wherever it leads.

Laughing Buddha

This time it was in the bones. Having survived two forms of cancer, including a melanoma, which is frequently deadly, my mother was a cancer veteran.

When she and Dad had called me several years earlier with news about the melanoma, their optimistic words didn't hide the timbre of terror behind them. I'd been more sanguine—a naive it-can't-happen response, rather than prescience. But in fact, it hadn't happened. Not then.

This time, I sensed, was different. Mom, who'd always been vigorous, now at eighty-one suddenly, surprisingly, had grown frail. I wasn't prepared for it. Small tasks required planning, and they exhausted her. Making carrot-raisin salad, sitting on her tall stool at the sink, was a morning's accomplishment. She marveled at my energy and often urged, "Honey, slow down," forgetting that she used to do as much.

The morning after my arrival in St. Louis in March 1996, we had an appointment with the oncologist. Braced against this meeting, Mom and I sat side by side, rigid in our chairs. Across from us behind his big desk, which seemed emblematic of the distance that stretched between us, Dr. Anderson confirmed what we'd already been told. Although Mom's was a rapidly progressing form of cancer, chemotherapy would give her an even chance for cure. He made it clear, however, that if the chemo regimen weren't completely successful, she would relapse. Then, further treatment, though available, would be painful and unlikely to succeed.

I looked at Mom as he talked. Her stoic exterior covered a frozen interior, I was sure. I slid my arm around her shoulders and found her body unyielding. In the clutch of brand-new shock, she was unable to accept the comfort I was trying to offer.

Next to large, blindless windows that ran the length of the office, on a long, low marble sill by the desk was a wooden statue of a Buddha. It was a laughing Buddha, with a beggar's sack slung over his shoulder and a round, protruding belly. My mind drifted to that laugh. I could almost hear it—clean, free of burdens and fears. I wondered how many people could laugh like that as they sat in the chairs we were sitting in and faced that formidable block of a desk. "Few, if any," I thought. "Most must have been like us. Scared. Just expressing it in different ways." So much dread, thick and dark, churning through the room, swirling around that wooden Buddha. . . .

Yet its presence seemed to me a blessing. This little statue was right where it belonged. In the midst of the tornado, it was a bright reminder of what's possible, of what's true, of the inner freedom awaiting each of us, if we choose to find it. For freedom is there, even amidst wall-to-wall fear. I knew it, not because

I had attained freedom, but because I'd had enough glimpses that I didn't doubt its existence.

At the moment, however, I was afraid. More than that, I was displaced. Wrenched from the monastery with little warning, my body was sitting in a chair in a doctor's office in a hospital in St. Louis, a city I hadn't lived in for twenty-five years. I wasn't sure where my mind was. And I didn't try to find out—floating with events was enough for now.

Mom and I had an assignment when we left the office. We needed to decide if she would undergo chemo or let the disease take its course. The decision was finally hers, but she wanted to reach it with my support.

First, however, lunch. As we drove home, we decided that we wouldn't decide yet. We would attend to our more urgent hunger. Besides, we needed a break from hard things.

I fixed lunch while Mom went into the half-bath near the kitchen. Washing lettuce for our cheese sandwiches, I heard muffled sounds from the bathroom. At first I thought she'd found a place alone to cry. But when she came out, her body was shaking with laughter. She explained in gasps, "You know what I was just doing? I was washing my hands, so I won't catch some disease!"

We sat down at the kitchen table, and we both laughed. Not the laugh of an awakened Buddha who has leapt beyond fear, but the laugh that momentarily releases tension, a giddy laugh, the laugh of little buddhas who someday—maybe—would learn how to find their freedom.

Finding Wisdom in Folding Laundry

I rode into town at high noon on March 1, 1996, astride a white horse, erect in posture, bearing a banner. I was on a mission: I was going to support my mother as she faced the diagnosis of cancer. Emblazoned on the banner in gold letters were the words, "I shall try to help my mother gain deeper insight into the transience of life and enable her to face death with greater acceptance." It was a big banner! It was no mean mission.

Buddhists are something like experts on dying. The *Tibetan Book of the Dead* isn't an isolated treatise in Buddhism. Much of Buddhist teaching guides a practitioner toward understanding the significance of death as a reality which, if deeply accepted, can transform life and imbue it with a profound ease. Death in Buddhist teaching, however, often refers not only to bodily demise but also, more subtly, to the death of the ego. The ego, that which causes us to rigidly identify with "my way" and "mine," mires us in emotional and intellectual stickiness, and it keeps us from true freedom. We need to learn to hold our lives, and all the people and things in it, lightly, with an open hand and a heart of loving kindness and respect.

Although I didn't pretend to be a master of this profound subject, I did assume, as I rode into St. Louis, that my years of spiritual training gave me an edge over my mother. It didn't occur to me that this attitude was arrogant. Nor did I realize, on a more practical level, that this preconceived notion was about to cloud my perception of what was really happening.

I didn't plan to preach from a pulpit or to try to convert my mother to Buddhist views. Nothing so coercive and unrefined. But I had a conviction—one I still contend with—that it's possible to share the wisdom of spiritual practices and insights, as I understand them, in a sensitive way that is readily accessible to non-Buddhists. I knew that there is a subtle balance between appropriate sharing and offensive pushing, and I didn't intend to fall into offense. What I wanted to do, to begin with, was to help my mother, who disliked talking about unpleasant subjects, express her feelings about this potentially fatal disease.

After initial hesitation and intense discussion between us, Mom decided to take chemotherapy. The decision kept us busy. We needed to schedule appointments for the next five months, educate ourselves about her disease, and learn about potential reactions to the chemo and measures to take in the event of reactions. And there were the daily doings—tidying the house, grocery shopping, cooking, washing. Because Mom wanted to do as much of this as she could manage, my role was to assist her where needed and undertake tasks she couldn't perform. Laundry was one of our joint projects. With my presence in the house, the load was double, and together, we sorted socks and tee shirts. We developed a routine for folding sheets: she held one end, and I backed up, holding the other so that the sheet didn't touch the floor; then we met in the middle with the folded product, all the while talking about the small activities of the day. Either of us could easily have done the job alone, but Mom clearly relished the companionship. And so did I. We had plenty to do and plenty to talk about.

What my mother didn't talk about, however, was dying, and that worried me. Did she fear death so much that she was avoiding the subject, as if it were a brooding castle deep in a forest that since childhood she'd been told was haunted and had been warned to stay away from? "She wouldn't be the first," I concluded.

I tried to skillfully give her a chance to discuss it. I didn't blurt out at the dinner table as we were eating, "Are you afraid to die? Let's examine this." No, I did it subtly. In a conversation about a film we'd just watched, I segued to the observation that the star's end was harder because he and his wife hadn't openly discussed his physical condition and their emotional reactions to it. There was no comment from Mom. I opened the way as I pulled up pansies, which were about to be killed by the summer heat, by commenting on the fragility of life. Our daily activities gave me many opportunities to touch the subject naturally. All to no avail.

I knew that real communication happens more readily when one opens a door for another from within a familiar room, rather than thrusting the other out into unknown territory, where he or she is likely to stand quivering or run for cover. And I knew that a person needs to choose whether to step outside, just glance through the doorway, or turn away.

With insistent cheer, Mom turned away. "All my subtlety lost in her pleasantries and chirpiness," I lamented. It was not only worrisome; I sensed a sham. I projected onto my mother expectations rooted in my own inner dynamics. In her place, I'd have talked about dying; not to would have felt fraudulent.

I fretted over the matter for months, worrying that I was being clumsy. "If only I could find the right words at the right time, then maybe she'd talk." I was convinced my mother harbored fears that were festering in her silence. I assumed that the words I needed existed somewhere, words that would pierce her resistance and allow her fears to flow freely, thereby lightening her affliction. In my zeal, I even tried the head-on "do you want to talk about dying?" approach.

I never found the right words or time because, it turned out, fear wasn't the issue. I later discovered that, in opting for chemotherapy, Mom had made a commitment to living. In her disciplined way, she was directing her energy toward coming out on the winning side of her fifty-fifty chance at survival. Discussing her fears, dwelling on the possibility of losing her battle, would have eroded her determination. Instead, she declared many times, like a mantra, "I've beaten this disease twice. I'll beat it a third time, too."

"I think you can do it, Mom," I responded, supporting her without recognizing the implications of her statement.

A year later, however, when there was no longer a point in struggling and when she'd begun to talk about death occasionally, Mom inadvertently explained her reticence. We were standing at the window passing binoculars between us for a hair-by-hair view of four deer that frequented the yard. Watching one of the youngsters butt the other with phantom antlers, forehead to forehead, she commented, "Look at them play, like they're fighting!" Then, in one of those obscure connections that enliven real talk, she added, "When I was trying to beat it last year, I had to stay optimistic because otherwise I couldn't keep up the fight."

At the time I took her remark as guileless, devoid of recognition that she'd just resolved a long worry for me. Later, however, I wondered if she hadn't been aware of my concern all along. Maybe each time I thought I was being subtle, she was thinking, "Oh no, there she goes again! Enough already!"

My polite mother had never said a word in rebuke. On the other hand, she hadn't explained either. A sentence from her might have helped me drop my effort and my worry.

Although at the time, I didn't understand why Mom didn't talk about dying, I eventually realized she wasn't going to do it. Many failed efforts taught me, finally, to give up trying to help my mother *my* way and to relax into helping *her* her way.

Such a simple lesson! It's one I thought I'd learned years before, but here it was again. In the guise of these new circumstances, it took me months to recognize it. Shifting perspective wasn't easy. It meant a little insult to my ego, a crimp in its style. I had to be willing to see beyond the fortress of my views and emotions and to accept that Mom's approaches had validity for her. When the chips are down, when teachings come off of a page of scripture and into real life, how many of us really welcome them? Being right is much more gratifying.

I was learning, not for the first time, that life is truer than missions. That it was enough to talk about the simple things we were talking about, to do the simple things we were doing. These things clearly made Mom happy, and they supported her. Each holding her ends of the sheet, coming together in the middle, we folded a lot of laundry.

We're a Team

"I'm a little scared," I confided to the chief resident, who was standing with me in a hospital corridor in midtown St. Louis.

That was an understatement! My insides felt welded solid. My mother, who'd been hospitalized for the past month, was about to be released. Someone would have to care for her, and my insides weren't ready for the job. "Wait! I'm just visiting. I'm not here to stay," I rebelled silently.

But here I was in St. Louis, in January 1997, about to care for my dying mother. My sister Gail, with a husband and career, had obligations in Los Angeles, while I, who was living in a monastery, was without obligations in the sense the world usually understands them. When we'd learned a few days earlier that Mom was terminally ill, I'd made my choice.

Actually, I'd been making it all along. I knew intuitively that my mother's sudden symptoms, which had reappeared while I was visiting, were linked to the cancer that lurked in her bones. The doctors needed proof, and that was a few weeks in coming. But I knew. Just as I knew what my decision would be. In a sense, it was no decision at all. It was simply a "yes" to the obvious.

When I wasn't numb at the prospect, I felt like a leaf, a crumbly fall leaf, caught in a whirlwind and wildly pitched about. When I'd left Mom five months earlier after the chemotherapy had ended and returned to the Abbey, I'd assumed that her cancer would recur, but I wasn't really prepared for it. In the vertigo of events of the past few weeks, three things were clear: Mom was going to die. I loved her. And being with her was exactly where I needed to be.

When I told Mom that I'd stay, she was quiet for a minute; then she urged me to return to my life. It was large-hearted statement on the face of it, and behind the face of it, even larger, because my mother deeply disapproved of my monastic choice. With a simple "thank you," she would have ensured that she could continue to live at home and that I would be diverted, at least temporarily, from a future she considered objectionable.

Her other option had been some sort of nursing facility. Stuck under a magnet on her refrigerator was an ad from a local paper: "Margaret's Loving Care—a nice change from a nursing home." Like most of the whatnots residing under the flower magnets there, it looked like a long-term inhabitant. Although she'd said little about it, Mom clearly knew that someday she might need an arrangement more supportive than what her solitary life provided. The prospect of leaving her home appalled her. But, being practical and independent-minded, she was considering her options. The lone nonflower magnet on the refrigerator read, "When the going gets tough, the tough get going." She wanted to make her own decisions rather than becoming a hapless recipient of circumstances. Maybe Margaret's Loving Care would have been her choice.

But I was firm. I was staying, and Mom was relieved and immensely grateful. Later on, I told her, and told her truly and often, that being with her was a two-way gift, a gift for me as well, but I think she didn't believe me.

At the beginning, however, as I stood in the hospital corridor and peered into the future, perceiving gifts in the situation was beyond my ability. I was simply responding to an inner voice that commanded "stay!"

Mom was overwhelmed by the life-changing news about her condition, by her sudden month in the hospital, and by an emergency operation on her knee to remove an acutely painful tumor. She had little energy left to notice my fear. I kept it close anyway, knowing this wasn't the time to discuss it with her, and feeling too overwhelmed to talk with anyone else. Silence was probably a mistake. I should have confided in friends, because fear grew in the silence like mold grows in a damp place. I was covered with it.

What did I know about taking care of a cancer patient? How long would I be called upon to do it, and how would I manage? Although I'd cared for her the preceding year during her chemotherapy, this was entirely different. This time she was going to die. It sounds obvious to say that that had never happened before, that in all my life my mother hadn't died. But the finality of it now was attention-stopping. It was real, and so was the fact that I was going to be a participant in the process.

"Maybe it'll be too hard, and I'll have to put her into a nursing home," I thought darkly. But even as I thought dark thoughts, I knew the answer to my fear, and that was another thing I knew for sure: step by step. I would manage from here to there, wherever, whenever "there" would be, by living step by step, in accordance with my spiritual training. The scripture recited in the Buddhist Lotus Ceremony contains the phrase "wandering in training one step at a time." I knew there was profound insight in this teaching, "one step at a time," but insight was for later. At the moment, as the phrase echoed in my mind, I reacted with a less-than-profound, "That's going to be me, all right, wandering and probably falling flat on my face daily!"

The chief resident at the hospital, Dr. Lyle, was reassuring. Responding to my admission that I was afraid, he patted my shoulder and said, "You'll do fine." On the deepest level, he was right, of course. I would do fine. I *was* fine. Even Mom was fine on the deepest level of truth where we are all pure expressions of That Which Is Deathless, the Eternal, God. But I didn't think Dr. Lyle was referring to the deepest level, and it was all the other levels that worried me.

So I procrastinated. Rather than discharging my mother from the hospital that week—it was already Thursday—I suggested to him that Monday would be better because . . . and I cited a good reason, but not the real one. He agreed. Monday it would be. I had the weekend, then, to adjust and plan for Mom's return.

A few days earlier, when Mom's condition had been diagnosed as terminal, we had been presented with the hospice option, and we took it. I had friends who were hospice volunteers, working with dying patients and their families. What little I knew about the organization was reassuring, but I'd never thought to be a recipient of their services. That was for other people. Maybe hospice was the kind of organization you could warm up to, but as I gazed down the corridor that afternoon, its too-happy colors turned dark. Like some nightmare, the bustle in the hall went hollow, and I couldn't see the end. Hospice seemed a flimsy thread to cling to.

Mom wanted to die naturally. "When it's time for me to go, I want to go," she had asserted more than once. Although she had completed a living will formalizing this desire years earlier, neither of us had realized that hospice's mission was just that. An international organization, hospice in America serves terminally ill people, helping them at home with medical care and emotional support. Hospice enables people to live the last phase of their life with quality and as little pain as possible, but without curative treatment or procedures that artificially prolong life.

Now, newly enrolled as a hospice patient, my mother was going to be visited two or three times a week by a nurse, who would be our contact for all her medical needs. I wouldn't have to call an array of doctors and wait for their responses; the nurse would talk with Mom's oncologist, who'd been designated her primary care physician, to determine medication to relieve her pain and discomfort.

There would be no more medical expenses either; hospice would pay them. We appreciated that benefit, even while we knew its real price was her life. Medical supplies would be delivered to the house, and a physical therapist would visit to help Mom regain use of her incapacitated knee. The alternative, clinic visits, would have meant my maneuvering her and

a heavy wheelchair into and out of the car and possibly nego-
tiating steps. Maybe I could have managed, but at that
moment, even walking back to my mother's bedside seemed
a task of uncertain outcome.

Learning that I could call hospice any time during the
ten thousand minutes of a week didn't halt my galloping fears,
as I stood in the hospital corridor, but I hoped it would help
slow them to a trot. Mom and I were both grateful for the range
of support. We knew this wasn't going to be easy.

Shortly before Mom was discharged, Dr. Lyle dropped by
her room. He urged us to call if we had questions and
offered each of us a business card.

"Oh, no," Mom said holding up a hand in stop position.
"One card between us is enough. We're a team."

It wasn't exactly a defining moment. The terms of our
situation were already frightfully clear to me. We were playing
on an unknown field with hospice as our coach, and—Mom had
said it well—we were a team.

Homecoming

Mom came home from the hospital in an ambulance on a stretcher and with a death sentence. I'd planned to bring her in the car, but when I got to the hospital, she was nauseated. She'd been vomiting for hours, or trying to, because now there was nothing left to bring up except sputum. Her leg was wrapped from ankle to thigh in a soft, foam-padded cast to protect her knee, which had just been operated on, and it couldn't be bent. Limp from the retching and the lack of food, she could barely squeak "hello."

The prospect of a car trip appalled me. Standing by her bedside, I envisioned it: not the front seat—she'd have to sit in the back, sideways, her leg straight on the seat, juggling barfbags and towels. Clearly it wouldn't work.

I arranged for an ambulance instead. None was available for an hour, and this was a relief, because, making a quick mental adjustment to my plans, I figured I'd have time to pick up her medicine from the pharmacy before she arrived. In her condition, I didn't want to leave her alone at home.

Kissing her on the cheek, I said, with my lips mimicking a smile, "I'll go to Dierbergs to get your medicine, and I'll be there to meet you when you get home, Mom."

She nodded weakly. At that moment her misery was her world. The transporting of her body was a mere outer event that little concerned her.

Walking out of the hospital that afternoon, I was different from the person who had walked in an hour earlier. Up until then, I'd been helping my mother, and although she'd been very sick at times, I'd had the unreasoned sense that it was merely a temporary indisposition and that I was pitching in until she was up on her own again. Now, blooming within was the blind responsibility of motherhood. I, who'd never been a mother, suddenly had become one, responding to that maternal imperative, that biological dictate, with which there is no arguing. Nothing was going to keep me from this task! My child-mother needed me and, to begin with, I was going to have her medicine for her when she got home. That sense of responsibility didn't leave me until the day Mom died.

The sudden flowering of motherhood did not, however, allay my doubts. "How am I going to manage this?" The question had been assailing me for days. As I drove down the interstate from the city to the pharmacy in the suburbs, four or five prescriptions in my purse along with careful notes on when to dispense them, I felt besieged.

"Calm down," I instructed. "This is going to work somehow. There's going to be a tomorrow. And a next day."

I wasn't sure about a day after that. I offered up a quick and earnest prayer; then I tried to focus on my driving. This was my spiritual practice: to give my attention to what was at hand, which is another way of saying, right now, to just drive. For if I allowed my mind to dwell on my fears about what might happen later, I'd be only partly aware, only partly awake to the present; the rest would be phantoms, empty and dread-filled "what ifs," and I, the haunted house they inhabited.

"Foot on the brake and stop, a little close to the red Corolla. Slow acceleration, moving to the inner lane, space between the pickup and black car, go—'What's it going to be like at home?'" Worry intruded. With effort, I brought my attention back to what needed to be done. "Merging left, there now, left-turn lane, blinker, stoplight ahead, but I'll make it through, now slowing, slowing . . . no oncoming traffic, turn here. Stop."

"We have all these." The pharmacist pointed to the prescriptions and checked them off, writing the name of a generic equivalent on one. "But we don't have this," he said, indicating the Duragesic patch. "It's a controlled substance and we'll have to order it. It'll take a couple of days."

The patch was the most important one, a narcotic that would enable my mother to endure her cancer pain as well as the pain in her knee, which was in the first stage of healing. "She's wearing a patch already, and maybe it'll last a day or two. But what if it doesn't?" I fretted silently.

"Okay. I don't see that there's any choice," I replied with resignation. And I thought, "A *bad* beginning. Is it always going to be so hard to get her medicine?"

I tried. Within the limit of the law, I tried to get home as fast as I could, but when I pulled up, the ambulance was already there. At the sight of that emergency vehicle parked in our driveway at the top of the hill, the lead hand that was squeezing my lower belly grabbed my heart. Mom, who was already on a gurney with two attendants maneuvering, asked weakly, "Where've you been?"

I wanted to protest, to say that the ambulance was the one who hadn't lived up to its side of the deal; it had come too soon. Instead, I simply said that I'd had to pick up her medicine first. Behind my comment was a sudden recognition that she must have been anxious, arriving home and not finding me there. My first venture into motherhood, and I'd let her down!

Resourceful even in sickness, Mom stated, "You weren't here, so I told them where we hide the key," and nodded toward the attendants who were preparing to roll her to the door.

In through the garage they wheeled her, through the adjoining room, the room where she would die six months later, then to the narrow hall leading to the rest of the house and to her bedroom at the other end. No luck. The hallway was too narrow to let the gurney through. Like a movie running in reverse, the attendants backed again into the room adjoining the garage, then through the garage, and onto the driveway.

Their next assault was at the front door, the gurney aimed like a battering ram. The sharp right turn from the foyer to the hall leading to my mother's room gave them problems. A second try was in progress when, suddenly, in the middle of the kitchen appeared a policeman. Where did he come from?

"Is everything all right here, folks?" he asked as the ambulance attendants were repositioning. He explained that someone had pressed the emergency alarm. I looked at the alarm button on the wall by the door and then at the gurney, which

I suspected to be the offender.

"Well, officer," I said, "my mother is just coming home from the hospital. She's feeling awful, and she's a new hospice patient. Aside from that, everything's okay." I decided to spare him the story about how okay I was.

We'd been home about an hour, Mom still retching, when the hospice pharmacy called. A carrier was on her way to the house to deliver Mom's medications, even the patch.

"Of course! Hospice!" In the torrent of new things that flooded this day of homecoming, I'd forgotten that hospice would deliver Mom's medications.

"Oh, thank you!" My voice surged with gratitude and relief. "Can you bring the medicine, and I'll get the prescriptions for you another time?"

I explained my mistake and my dilemma. I didn't want to leave my mother alone while I returned to the store to retrieve the prescriptions. But the pharmacy was firm. Without the prescriptions, they couldn't deliver the medicine. It was law.

I propped Mom up with pillows. By her side on her big double bed, I placed containers, towels, tissues, a damp washcloth—everything she might need for vomiting in the next thirty minutes.

"I'll just be gone a little while, Mom. So don't worry."

The trip to Dierbergs was a little easier this time. Hospice was there to support us.

Step by Step

The day before my mother came home, I stood in her room and made a mental check. From a friend, a full bouquet, featuring five large and fragrant Casablanca lilies, which I'd placed on the highboy across from her bed to welcome her home. Fresh linens and a cleaning, a once-over-for-principle's-sake, since Mom's room was always tidy. With its northern exposure, hers was the coldest room in the house—all right for nighttime sleeping curled under a comforter, but now, returning from the hospital, she would have to live there until she healed enough to resume, temporarily, a more normal routine. So I'd bought a small space heater, which I'd placed on the night table. It could direct a flow of heat straight on, or oscillate and hug her in a wedge of warmth. And on the bed, a king-sized bed she and my father had shared, an extra blanket, just in case.

Because trips to the bathroom would be an ordeal, with the pain in her knee and her leg in a cast, I'd stationed nearby a borrowed commode, and next to that, to hold the toilet paper, an old-fashioned muffin stand that had adorned a corner in the living room, displaying knickknacks. It was a comedown in stature but more practical, for sure. Even after her knee had healed, I knew that commode and little muffin stand would be part of our lives.

Then there were the usual small supplies—pillows, newspapers, a *Time* magazine. Towels. A box of tissues. And a small steel bell to ring when she needed me, the kind used at shop counters with a button in the middle to tap for service. Next to her on the bed, I'd placed a "grabber," a yard-long metal device with a pincher at the end, which had been recommended by hospital staff so without moving she could pick up things within its reach. (We later discovered it wasn't as useful as it looked.)

All of this was standard sickroom stuff, but I stood back and appreciated it anyway. "At least the room is ready for her," I thought cheerlessly, feeling I wasn't.

I was right. Her first hours at home the next afternoon unnerved me. Lying in that bed wasn't simply my mother. It was a Hospice Patient, a person with terminal cancer who'd been removed from the care of nurses and aides and orderlies and technicians and doctors, all with their routines and paraphernalia, complex and simple, an endless supply—from an environment of total professional support, to me and our commode and our little steel bell to signal an emergency. I hadn't slept well the night before, anticipating her arrival.

Standing before her, I felt gawky. I didn't know where to put my hands or how far away from the bed to stand. My body felt as strained as when I'd first perched on the triangular patch of a two-wheeler's seat, stretching to reach the handlebars and the pedals far below, struggling to fit myself into the new position. At the time, Dad had been there to catch me when I lost my balance. Now, no one was. The sense of reassurance conferred by hospice support that had embraced me the preceding afternoon proved fleeting. Aside from Mom and me, the planet now felt uninhabited.

The first thing I hadn't prepared for was her nausea. I quickly arranged containers, three of them, so she could hold one while I washed the other out. The third was our reserve. To clean and refresh her face, I folded a damp washcloth in a bowl, which would keep the bedding from getting wet.

The nausea made her mouth dry and sour. "A little Coke will fix that," I suggested.

Searching the refrigerator, I found only diet Coke—not a calorie of nutritional value. I seldom drink soda, and my mother, always conscious of her calories, drank only the artificially sweetened kind. "Okay, put Coke—the real thing—on the shopping list. And Seven-Up too." Later, our hospice nurse recommended Gatorade, which has electrolytes to restore a body's depleted supply, but at the moment Gatorade was beyond my ken.

I filled a glass with the calorie-less Coke, a plastic glass in case she dropped it, and I prided myself on this bit of foresight. Propped in bed and weak, Mom tried to tilt the glass to her lips. "I could use a straw, please," she whispered, careful to say "please."

Back in the kitchen, I found paper straws with a crinkle near the top for bending. "Well, that's smart," I thought, looking kindly on the straws I'd never bothered to think about before. I felt a surge of warmth for whoever invented them and for Mom at having a supply on hand. At the moment no blessing was too insignificant for my gratitude.

Although she took only a few sips, they were too much; the Coke came up. I had a container ready. Step by step, I was learning: real soda, in a plastic glass, with a bendy straw, and only a little at a time because I'd probably have to throw it out anyway. And always on hand, a container for vomiting.

"You need to try to eat, Mom, just a little. You can't have an empty stomach," I advised later, sounding more knowledgeable than I felt.

"Why can't she have an empty stomach? The hospital discharged her that way," I argued with myself. But I stood firm— it was only common sense. I didn't know how long it would go on, this vomiting, but sooner or later she could die of dehydration and exhaustion. I had to offer her something, and I hoped that by the time I brought the food, her stomach would be less hostile. Solid food wasn't an option, of course. But jello, that first choice for sick folks, was worth a try.

The copper flour canister in the pantry held several boxes of jello. All calorie-less, I discovered as I laid them out on the kitchen counter. Another item for the shopping list—real jello. "So it's bouillon then," I concluded aloud. I was aware I was using the sound of my voice like a cane, to steady myself, to serve as a hedge against what I really wanted to do, which was to run out of the house and cry.

I was overwhelmed by a sense that Mom and I were adrift, alone in a small boat with no help in sight, and I was doing the rowing. Already, just three hours after her return, I wanted to be back on dry land. I wouldn't have abandoned ship, even if I'd had the chance, but I longed to. The rowboat image stayed with me during our next six months, as we drifted closer and closer to the edge. . . .

Contacting hospice didn't occur to me that first day because I was too new to remember they were a resource for just such occasions. And also because a hospice nurse was due to visit the next day, and I assumed that we had to wait. And most of all, I didn't call hospice because doctors and nurses at the hospital had told us that Mom's nausea was normal. It was a typical reaction to her new medication. "It usually takes a few days for the body to adjust," a nurse had assured us. In the meantime, I was to give her medication to settle her stomach.

The trouble was, the Compazine wouldn't stay down any more than the Coke or bouillon had. Even in suppository form, the medication had no effect. She retched all that first night, and she rang the bell often, with many apologies. By the next morning, we were two exhausted sailors in that boat.

Before Mom had come home, I had considered a hiring private-duty nurse's aide. "Be kind to me," I'd counseled myself. "Even if we don't need her, it would be nice to have someone else here at the start. I could always let her go."

"Step by step," another voice countered. "Don't try to pre-think what you can't know. Take it as it comes, one step at a time. Go on from there—the clean approach."

Here it was again: "wandering in training one step at a time." That phrase from the Lotus Ceremony that I'd recited many times in the past was instructing me now. I listened, grateful for the guidance. It was like a handrail along a slippery path.

The first night clearly answered the question. I couldn't be nurse both day and night. Not in the long run I couldn't.

L ee was a fine nurse—with squeaky shoes. As she walked in and out of my mother's sickroom the second night, the squeaking kept me awake, but I was too tired and depressed to get up and ask her to take the shoes off. By the next morning, I realized that squeaky shoes or not, a nurse in the house and the little ringing bell would keep me awake unless I moved to a room farther from the activity.

The only sensible choice was the room off of the garage. Without carpet or a table lamp, it sometimes served as my mother's office. "She must use it only during daylight hours," I'd thought, speculating on how she worked in the gloom of two tiny wall lamps and a ceiling light of negligible effect. Most of all, however, the room was a place to walk through, to and from the garage, and a storage room of sorts.

There would be problems with this new room. The ranch-style house wasn't designed for well people and very sick ones at the same time; the only room for nursing aides to sit in was near the garage room, which meant I would need to wear earplugs at night. My chances of sleeping, however, were better there than in my old room, which was near Mom's. The prospect was depressing, because I liked my bright back room. It was my sanctuary, and the new arrangement would mean I'd have to live between both, with some inconvenience.

I started planning my move, but I didn't get far because of the hospital bed.

Before Mom had come home, I had decided to keep her bed rather than renting a hospital bed. "She's slept in it for years, most of them with Dad, and now she's been given a death notice. She needs as much emotional support as she can get," I'd reasoned. The comfort of coming home to her familiar room, bed and all, seemed to me more important than anything a hospital bed might do for her. If we needed one, I could rent it later.

Later was Thursday. In three days, Mom knew that the pillows and the propping didn't work. Her back, her neck, her shoulders, all over she was sore. But I didn't regret my first decision about the bed. Not a bit. I was beginning to learn that I could relax with my choices and keep my balance. I was beginning to feel I might handle the situation after all.

Because *I* wasn't handling it. That was the paradox. Step-by-step was. The phrase was like some little being echoing within me—a being I could cotton up to, talk to, which maybe was an index to my sense of desperation. "Okay, Step-by-step, what now?" I'd ask. It seemed better than wailing and showing Mom how distraught I was.

Some people talk to God, the Eternal, and I did, too—all the time. Step-by-step was part of the dialogue. Maybe a good way to describe it is that Step-by-step felt like the operational face of the Eternal. When I got my fears and desires out of the way and simply listened softly, then Step-by-step guided me through the small details that needed attention. It showed me the best way to proceed.

Such listening wasn't a matter of hearing voices literally, of course. Nor did it mean I needn't organize. Moving aside the flower magnets and the "when the going gets tough" magnet,

I put a large magnetic pad on the refrigerator door listing the new phone numbers in our lives—hospice numbers and the private nursing service—as well Mom's medications and when to administer them. In a looseleaf binder I kept notes—questions to ask our hospice nurse, a schedule of visiting hospice support people, and a weekly schedule of the private-duty assistance I'd requested.

Organizing was useful. Moreover, it was comforting. It was our breadcrumb trail through this forest of new activity, not so much marking our way back as affirming that we were forging ahead with purpose.

Beyond that, Step-by-step showed me when it was pointless to prethink or organize, when organizing would just run me around with needless activity. It made priorities plain. It was practical. And I was amazed. I, who'd always thought myself fairly impractical, was discovering a sureness in practical matters I didn't know I possessed. Not an I-know-what-to-do-next kind of sureness, but an I'm-listening-and-I'm-willing-to-try. The trick was to trust Step-by-step and to keep my busybody personal agenda out of the way. The trick was to be still.

The hospital bed presented a logistical problem. The rental company wouldn't deconstruct Mom's big bed, which occupied most of her room, and she didn't want to wait until Gail and my brother-in-law Bruce, who'd be visiting soon, would arrive and help me with the effort. Step-by-step told me that we needed to get the hospital bed quickly and worry about moving it to her room later. There was only one available room, and that was the room off the garage, which I'd now furnished with a small rug and floor lamp in preparation for my own move.

When I brought Mom into the room, the hospital bed ready for occupancy, she exclaimed, "I like this room! I think I'll stay here. It's warmer than mine."

Having assumed that she wanted to die in her room, I wouldn't have asked Mom to move. Now that psychological comfort wasn't an issue, however, it was clear that this was the better arrangement, putting her closer to the nurses (who sat in the den until called, because Mom valued her privacy and didn't want them waiting in her room). And, once she was well enough to get up, she would be closer to the den and kitchen. Also, happy fact, I could stay in the back room, which would be quieter now, a good place for sleeping and meditating. Bless Step-by-step! There's no telling where it's going to lead. Except it's probably not where you expect.

Ode to Annie

"Who's Annie? Your mother's calling for Annie!" Rushing into the kitchen where I was fixing dinner, Maderia, a private nursing aide, exhaled the question in one urgent breath.

I raced to Mom's room and thrust into her hands a clear plastic container, tall and triangular, with liquid measures up the sides, the kind used in hospitals for urine and other liquid samples. She vomited into it.

When Mom was in the hospital, we had discovered the value of these containers. Larger than the low-sided kidney-shaped ones, these were perfect for vomiting. They were easy to hold, and they contained a serious amount of fluid. The plastic tended to crack if squeezed too hard, but why quibble when they were so useful when you needed them?

As Mom did. After three days of intestinal rebellion, a compassionate hospice nurse finally released her from the tyranny of the narcotic painkiller that was making her vomit. I think Mom would have rejoiced had she been strong enough.

Mom had used the larger containers in the hospital when she was nauseated, and we had talked about taking some of these useful items home with us, knowing she'd likely be nauseated again. We didn't know how soon.

Worth just a few cents each, the containers, which are but minor players in any daily hospital drama, became invaluable in our eyes. A generous nurse gave us four, but immediately upon arriving home, we cracked one. Three precious containers left then, to last the duration. We handled them like Waterford crystal. It didn't occur to us that we might get more. Those three did last, while the cracked fourth, bound with duct tape, became a bedside container for Mom's brushes and combs. Afterwards, I presented the three whole ones to our hospice nurse to pass on to someone else in need, but I think she didn't appreciate their value the way we did.

It was clear right away that we needed a name. Mom couldn't call out as she was on the verge of vomiting, "Plastic urine sample container, please!" By the time she'd uttered that mouthful, the container would have been superfluous. "Plastic container" was too impersonal; "barf box," too crude. "That thing" (pointing) was too vague.

"How about 'Annie'? It's simple and friendly," I suggested.

I was inspired by Annie, the female lead in *Sleepless in Seattle*. I'd rented the video an evening or two before Mom came home. Its sweet, light theme was a distraction, though a fleeting one, from the desolation that usurped my days.

I was meditating with desolation. I was trying to do one of the hardest things in the world. I was trying to pry my focus loose from the content of my drama, away from those thoroughly engrossing details that echoed in my mind like a voice in a series of canyons, and focus instead on the flow, the process of thinking. This is a place of mindful attention.

I couldn't do it. So overwhelming was the drama that time and again my attention got stuck in the thoughts. Eventually I gave up and turned to another technique. I found I could focus on how the drama felt in my body. I could observe its physical impact, noting the location (the heart, solar plexus, or elsewhere) and experiencing the feeling there (it was usually icy and heavy). The shift in attention located me in present time, in what was happening at that moment rather than in thoughts about the past or worries and doubts about the future. Reality exists only now. Right here.

When I accepted the glacier that encased me like a prehistoric mammal, when I focused on it quietly and didn't squirm to escape or become angry, a sense of contentment often arose. Contentment was right there in the ice pack. They were the same thing, but in different forms. And when the glacier rolled in again with all its frigid weight, as it did time after time, sometimes it was a little less hard to bear. Moreover, I noticed that even within the deepest freeze, there was physical change, however minute. A little icicle melted or, for a moment, the glacier disappeared altogether. Nothing is permanent.

Personalizing the plastic containers was another way of accepting desolation. Years earlier, I would have coped grimly. Girding my loins, gritting my teeth, and, with sword in hand, I'd have slogged on. Now—gift of my spiritual training—I was trying to befriend desolation by bringing something dear and playful to our situation.

The serenity prayer asks God to grant one the serenity to accept the things one cannot change, the courage to change what one can, and the wisdom to know the difference. I think "to accept *playfully* the things one cannot change" is better. Playful acceptance doesn't mean denying or trivializing anguish. It is an effort to find the light within it.

Once released from the patch, Mom recovered from her nausea. Then, we found that the round-the-clock doses of narcotics she'd been receiving had virtually eliminated her pain. For a while, she needed no medication at all. But pain returned soon enough, more intensely than before. And the nausea returned, too. At those times, like a child hugging a teddy bear, Mom often fell asleep with Annie nestled by her cheek.

Love at the Eleventh Hour

Troubles may come in threes, but twos was more than I thought I could handle. About the time Mom came home from the hospital with the diagnosis of terminal cancer, I got more bad news. It was about another relationship, and it was unexpected. Suddenly, I was facing not one, but two big losses, and I wasn't sure how I was going to cope.

As Mom slowly recovered from her nausea and her knee surgery, I wondered if I should share my new pain with her. I considered the good reasons why I shouldn't. "She's facing death. It's all so new, such a shock—a month in the hospital and now home for the last time. It's unfair to burden her with my problems, too." These were reasons enough to not tell her. But there was another reason, one I didn't put on my list, but which weighed as heavily as the others: I wasn't used to sharing my problems with my mother.

Unlike many people, I was lucky, or blessed with the good karma, to emerge from childhood unscarred by emotional issues concerning my parents. Ours had been an environment of love, and, in the way of children, I took it for granted. It was just how things were. However, although there were no emotional scars, there was a wall. We weren't close, and, as I grew past childhood, I stopped talking about "real problems" with my family. As a married adult living in the Washington, D.C., area, I usually began the weekly telephone conversation with my mother with the standard "Hi, Mom, how are you?"

"Fine. How are you?"

"I'm fine. I had a little cold, but I'm over it now. Anything new with you?" And so on. We always closed with an "I love you," and we meant it. It was comforting to know Mom was there, that she was getting along fine, and that she loved me. I think she was similarly comforted. Except, of course, I wasn't always fine. I'm sure she wasn't either.

I remember having lunch with her in a dainty tearoom on a winter afternoon during one of my periodic visits to St. Louis years earlier. Although I'd soon be in the midst of a divorce, I kept my comments light. "This quiche is wonderful. Do you think they give away the recipe?" I had an agenda for when I'd tell her my news, and it wasn't yet. So I drew the warmth of the tearoom and our sunny conversation around me like a blanket, and I kept at bay the turmoil that lay just ahead.

Mom was no paradigm of openness either. Operating on the "if you can't say something nice, don't say it" principle, she seldom discussed her problems with me, or with anyone, as far as I know. Maybe she thought problems weren't nice. Nor did Dad readily discuss personal issues, though he was more emotional in expression. I suspected their reticence was generational, an orientation so unlike my own. As a teenager, I had talked with girlfriends on the phone for hours, microscopically examining the states of our psyches with regard to the *real* issues in our lives, which usually meant boys.

Living with Mom during her final illness, I gradually learned that her optimistic exterior wasn't simply the evasion I'd thought it to be, that she was dealing with issues in her way, and I grew to respect her courage.

Nonetheless, I found her unwavering optimism irritating at times. One morning soon after I'd first come to live with her in 1996, I walked into the den, which we called the sitting room, to say good morning. Greeting me from her yellow chair, she chirped, "Good morning, Rosebud."

Rosebud? The origin of the name was a mystery to me. Whatever its significance, I certainly didn't feel like a Rosebud. Having recently learned that Mom had only an even chance of survival if she underwent chemotherapy, and still in shock over my abrupt transition from monastic to St. Louis life, I wasn't sleeping well at night. Now I had just finished my morning meditation, and my "good morning" response, as I walked into the room, contained a mix of several reactions.

Sometimes her forced optimism was humorous. On vacation in Florida years earlier, after Dad had died, Mom and I took a day trip to the Everglades. I drove, while she wielded the map. From Sanibel Island where we were staying, down Alligator Alley, we came to an unclearly marked turn. "Right," we decided, guided more by instinct than by reason. A half hour later, with gas running low and the sky growing dense with thunderheads, we found ourselves on a desolate two-lane road passing the grounds of a prison that seemed to go on forever. Mom was cheerful.

Peering at the gas gauge, she said brightly, "We still have an eighth of a tank of gas, and Everglades City should be coming up soon."

Several minutes later, we saw a woman walking with a baby by the roadside in the gloom. When this improbable and most welcome apparition confirmed we were on the right road, Mom and I giggled with relief. Thanking her and driving on, I turned to Mom and we confessed what neither of us had admitted before: "I was scared."

Mom took her cheery reserve into her final illness. Saying only the necessary minimum about how she was feeling, she would typically comment, "I'm a little nauseated. Would you please bring me a Compazine?" This, usually when the situation had reached a point of no return.

I kept urging her, gently I hoped, to be more open. It became a project of mine. "You know, Mom, you need to tell me how you're feeling so we can get you relief as soon as possible."

I tackled the emotional factor, too. "It's natural to be upset by all this. Anybody would be. Talking about it can help, and I want you to know, I'm here if you want to talk. You won't be bothering me. Really."

Although my advice had no noticeable effect, seeing that advice in print did. A booklet for hospice patients, given to us by our nurse Barbara, stressed that talking with loved ones and caregivers about one's pains and fears is critical to a patient's physical and emotional well-being.

Mom mulled it over. One morning in her easy chair, she pointed to the booklet and said, "It says here that a hospice patient needs to tell the primary caregiver what's going on. So

I want to tell you something I haven't been saying. . . ."

It was a beginning, and although she retained considerable reserve until she died, Mom slowly began to be a bit more open. She began to talk a little more honestly about her pain and sometimes, infrequently, even about her emotional reactions.

I welcomed her greater openness with me, but I had reservations about the reverse. Sharing my bad news now would reveal my vulnerabilities. It would breach a virtual law of my universe, for it would mean I was turning to my mother for comfort. That hadn't been part of my plans when I came to St. Louis. I wanted the rules of our relationship to change one way, but I'd never considered a two-way change. I hadn't considered a true mutuality where, in addition to giving love to Mom in her hurt place, I would receive it in mine. Even at this eleventh hour, when my mother had returned from the hospital with a terminal diagnosis, I wasn't sure I was ready for that kind of love from her.

Besides the fact that I was unpracticed at confiding in my mother, another reservation constrained me. Two of the four Noble Truths that the Buddha discovered from his training, and which countless others have discovered from theirs, are that the source of suffering is attachment, and that the way to free ourselves from suffering is to free ourselves from attachment. Practitioners struggle long and deeply with these truths, often with a sense of revulsion. For, at one level of understanding, they seem to mean we shouldn't love anyone or anything. That notion is an affront to one of our sweetest human instincts. This initial understanding (actually misunderstanding) can lead you to feel guilty about loving and even to efforts to back away from or—using a more austere term—to renounce what you love. People who have trained for years can still have misunderstandings.

I did. I thought I'd already worked to a deeper insight into the nature of nonattachment, but the weight of misunderstanding pulled at me now: by sharing honestly with Mom, I would be opening myself to new vistas of love. I had to remind myself, as I waged my debate, that at a deeper level, nonattachment means honoring love as a beautiful and natural human expression. Simultaneously, it means recognizing that love must be given with an open hand. Nonattached love means loving without grasping, without trying to possess what one loves.

The problem with possessiveness is, first of all, it doesn't work. The "Dear Abby" columns in the newspaper testify to that. Moreover, possession presupposes fixed entities—a subject who possesses and an object that is possessed. The concept is based on a limited view of who we really are. We cannot possess anyone or anything, nor can we be possessed, because the "we," the "I," that seems so solid is a mirage. There is no self present in the ordinary sense, to do the possessing. While this statement outrages everyday understanding, its meaning begins to become visible as one practices with clearer awareness. On every level of existence—from the gross, exterior events of life to the submolecular physical and subtle mental levels, there is continual change. What exists one instant no longer exists the next. Our boundaries are shifting and permeable. We are interrelated with all that is.

One morning, I sat on Mom's bed, and I shared my pain with her. I cried and she cried. Then, hugging me, this woman who was facing death said, "Up to now what has happened to me is unimportant. What you're telling me now is important. I love you."

I doubt that Mom sensed my struggle to speak from that deeper place of honesty. But her own words were, and will always remain, a gift of unutterable value—an expression, at the eleventh hour, of a lifetime of love.

Hames and Bopeep

In what must rank as one of the great UpWords moves of all time, my mother, placing four letter-tiles on the gameboard, stacking two of them on existing words, created four new words, down and across, and scored thirty-two points. She sat back with a small, satisfied smile.

"Wow!" I exclaimed. "How did you do that?"

We were in the midst of our favorite board game, which, as long as she was able, we played a couple of times a week. So many historic moves. In an opening turn, I once gained twenty bonus points by using all seven tiles to form one word. "We'll never have another 'bedroll'," we declared after that.

There were also nonmoves that won't find a place in the UpWords chronicles, but were just as memorable.

"How about 'Bopeep'?" Mom asked hopefully, tiles poised for placement, eliding the double name into a single word.

"Nope, it's a proper name. It's against the rules," I replied.

A game or two later she happily began to dig herself out

of a tight spot by forming "Tarzan." I nixed the move: "Same as 'Bopeep'. Can't be done."

"You are *so* mean!" she laughed, withdrawing her tiles.

Any activity, no matter how pleasurable, has its contrary side. Pleasure and displeasure, happiness and suffering are tightly interlinked. Every longing that blossoms into fulfillment contains seeds of discontent. In our UpWords games, the contrary side appeared in the competitiveness of the sport. Although we began each game benignly—we wanted to enjoy ourselves and allow each other to do so—as our game history lengthened, we inevitably felt the cut of competition.

When I won too many times in a row, Mom's enthusiasm waned, and she didn't want to play for a week or two. That was no fun. More important, it defeated the game's main purpose as far as I was concerned, which was to help promote her sense of well-being.

The remedy was simple: let her win. But carefully, for my mother was sharp, and, had she suspected, she likely would have found a wired game a greater affront than a string of losses.

Letting Mom win was simple enough in theory, but, oh, the lure of a good move! It pulled at me in spite of myself. "Just this one move . . . I'll think about fudging the rest later," I temporized many times.

Losing by design had another pitfall—smugness. I was quietly smug, of course, nothing crass, but inwardly I preened in the glow of virtue.

I preened, that is, until Mom won all on her own, which

happened often enough. "Wait a minute!" I thought. "She's not supposed to win this one; this is *my* game!" Though I hadn't played UpWords before arriving in St. Louis, I now found myself caught by two sticky little attachments—good moves and controlling behavior. Here was Buddhism 101! Attachment is the cause of suffering. We attach to things and suffer when we can't have them, or we fear losing them once we do have them. The two attachments that I'd just acquired were minor enough, but they clearly made the point.

Finding profound significance in a mere game may seem to be a stretch, but as meditators learn, we can observe the relationship between attachment and suffering anywhere. It's there for the perceiving. A little funny, really, how it reaches right down into minutia. Once you start paying attention, nothing is off limits.

Over the months, Mom and I slowly developed our own UpWords rules. These evolved naturally, without contrivance. "Calvin-ball rules" we called them, after the shock-haired, six-year-old cartoon character with an electric personality whose only rule in ball playing was "make it up as you go along." Mom and I weren't as free-wheeling as Calvin, but our UpWords gradually transformed from a competitive sport to a cooperative one. Prolonged shifting of position in one's chair while deliberating a turn or grumbling about one's tiles were signals that Calvin-ball rules were in order. Then one of us would advise, scrutinizing the other's lineup of tiles, "You can get rid of your 'z' and 'y' if you put them here and here on 'lane' for 'zany'." That this tactic made scorekeeping irrelevant didn't stop us from tallying and from feeling very pleased when our tallies climbed over the two hundred mark, or complaining when they were low. It was a joint pleasure and a joint displeasure—altogether more satisfying than the old competitive outcomes. And it was much easier than the effort I'd been making to keep the winning balance right.

In this relaxed setting, Mom had one rule she seldom breached: she didn't like to use "dirty" words. If they're in the dictionary, they're legal according to the rulebook. But Mom used such words only in a pinch and then with apologies. "Pus" she spelled in one game after an apologetic preface. I thought the word unfortunate because it gave her only four points. She disliked it because, while it wasn't actually "dirty," it was unpleasant. Coaching from the sidelines, I tried to ease her way: "Go ahead, do it, Mom. It's okay." But I soon heard myself echoing her and apologizing as I formed the word "slut." I was relieved a turn or two later when I could change it to "slip."

UpWords was my mother's kind of amusement. She worked hard at her vocabulary. Her Webster's, with its broken spine and dust jacket cut from a brown paper bag, resided on a table next to her reading place. It spent more time with her than any other book or, for that matter, any human being after Dad died. So when Mom could teach me a word, she was very pleased.

"Hame," she spelled one day in an UpWords game.

"What's a 'hame'?" I asked. I've been a horse lover since I was old enough to be placed on the back of a Shetland pony, led by a guide, who walked alongside holding the bridle. I probably know more about horses than many people, but I didn't know "hame" when Mom used it.

She defined it precisely. Reflecting a certain lack of confidence in her definition, I consulted her dictionary on the spot, and I found she was right. She was gracious enough not to express hurt over my doubt or to gloat that she had been vindicated. Thereafter, "hame" became one of our favorite game words.

Watching a video one evening after the dictionary incident, we noticed a horse in a street scene, plodding along drawing a cart. "There's a hame!" I exclaimed, pointing to the gear securing the traces. I was aware that I sounded like a five-year-old proudly showing teacher she'd learned her lessons. Because my dictionary arrogance was a still a sore memory for me, this felt like a chance to redeem myself. I was happy to sound like a five-year-old.

Birds of a Different Feather

"Is that Mary?" asked the cashier at the checkout counter at Wal-Mart, pointing to a photograph in my wallet. My wallet was open as I fished for money to pay for my purchases, inadvertently revealing a photograph that's a private reminder to myself. It is a photo of a painting of Avalokiteshwara, or Kwan Yin, the Buddhist embodiment of compassion.

"No," I replied. "It represents compassion and loving kindness. It's Buddhist."

Looking at me, her eyes like full moons, she exclaimed, "Are you a Buddhist? I've never seen an American Buddhist before!"

Suddenly, instead of being one more person in an anonymous line of people waiting to pay, I became a rare bird.

"I look pretty much like everybody else, don't I?" I objected, feeling my plumage was as ordinary as a sparrow's, no big deal.

"No," she replied earnestly. "You look like a Catholic."

She clearly meant it as a compliment. We laughed, and I, all the more heartily, because I'd been raised as a Jew.

I told this story about a week later when Barbara, our hospice nurse, was visiting. She and Mom also laughed. Then Mom asked, "Why didn't you tell me before?"

It was a good question—one I didn't answer, although I knew why. I hadn't told her because I wasn't sure how she would react. In Barbara's presence, the story came naturally. I intuitively felt that Barbara's response would be positive, and I hoped it would help Mom enjoy the story, too.

Mom and I had a history. I'd traveled far since my early twenties when I left Judaism. I was driven by a spiritual realization, an "awakening," I called it, that made Judaism, as I'd been taught it, incidental to my life. I struck out on my own, following this new level of awareness. At the beginning—which lasted years—I often blundered and was belligerent. In self-defense, of course—that's how I saw it—for I didn't realize that the threats I perceived to my new spiritual strivings were only in my mind. Not that there wasn't some opposition. But when one is centered, nothing is truly a threat. There is no need to justify or convince others. No need for words that glint like bayonets in sunlight. Centering is better than bayonets.

Raw and defensive, and either unsure where I was heading or sometimes too very sure, I regarded my family's reactions with hostility. I was closed and arrogant in turn.

Overall, my parents bore up with a sweet restraint that I didn't appreciate. I marvel at it now, though, and I'm grateful. Still, there were some rough times.

My parents, both raised in Orthodoxy, had evolved into "relaxed" Jews—they observed, but were far from practicing rigorously. Fairly conventional in their views, they had few tools with which to relate to what was calling to me. I'd become more open about my Buddhist spiritual practices around the time Dad died, and Mom was left to cope with that one without him. "My daughter, the Buddhist" was hard enough. "My daughter, the Buddhist monk" (for that was my aspiration now) was impossible.

"Why do you want to be a monk?" she asked many times. (The term "monk" is gender-neutral in the order that I wanted to join. Both men and women are called monks.) "Why not be a Buddhist without the monk part?"

I understood her dilemma. Monkhood isn't a standard occupational choice. And for a person raised in Judaism, which lacks a monastic tradition, it is especially hard to grasp.

There are times when words, no matter how clearly articulated, clarify nothing because the person they're spoken to isn't in a position to hear them openly. I was pretty sure this was so now. I was tempted to reply as had a musician who'd said in effect, when asked why he loved his music, "If you have to ask, I can't tell you."

True, perhaps, but with a bayonet. Bayonets aren't only fighting words, but sometimes simply hard ones, uttered with conceit or without compassion. Bayonets are words said with tight lips. Possibly, the person asking about music yearned to feel its pulse in his veins. Possibly, something in the musician's demeanor—a look in his eyes, the tilt of his head, a depth in his voice—would have opened the questioner's path to music in a way words couldn't. Possibly, if I explained, Mom would feel my answer.

I tried, but I think my lips were a little tight. And she tried. Maybe hers were, too. In the end, she said, "You're an adult.

And you'll do what you'll do. I don't understand it, but I want you to be happy."

Could I expect more?

Actually, there *was* more. A few years before her final illness, Mom and I talked about meditation. I explained that, while it is a basic Buddhist practice, no religious doctrine is involved in practicing it. Anyone can do it and benefit. Later, as a meditation teacher, I instructed people of various religious backgrounds, and most found that a regular mediation practice deepened them in their faith. Although I didn't explain this to my mother, she hadn't needed much convincing. She'd already heard about meditation as a stress reduction technique, and that seemed persuasive.

"Okay, I'll try," she agreed.

I instructed her, and, sitting in chairs, we began. A minute perhaps had passed when she announced, "I've got to stop. I'm getting dizzy."

"Wow!" I thought, "Something's happening!" I assumed that after only seconds of meditation, my mother was beginning to experience a deepening of awareness and, because she was unaccustomed to it, she mistook it for dizziness. I was impressed. Mom, however, was not, and the experience ended her meditation career. She had tried.

By the time I came to St. Louis to live with her, Mom and I had reached something of a balance. I think we both realized that focusing on our differences wouldn't serve any good purpose. No bayonets, not even little needles. We tried respect instead, which is what we'd really been trying to extend all along, but with only spotty success. Now, however, the dire circumstances seemed to make mutual respect easier to achieve.

For my part, I had matured enough in my spiritual training that I no longer felt threatened by my mother's choices and reactions, or by anyone else's, for that matter. I intended to support her every way I could, and that included participating in Jewish observances when appropriate. Years earlier, I would have found the prospect agonizing; now it was almost appealing.

I encouraged Mom to continue her activities at her Reform temple when she was able. Mom loved the book and political affairs discussion groups, Friday services, and talking politics with her friend, the rabbi. But chemotherapy stole her energy, and after several weeks away from temple, she hesitated to return because, always reticent about personal matters, she didn't want to explain her absences. In addition—the ultimate factor, one women readily understand—she was embarrassed to wear the wig she'd bought to cover her bald head.

Yet she longed to go. One Friday evening when the congregation was holding its usual potluck supper followed by a service and Mom was feeling fairly well, I urged her, "Go. You'll enjoy it."

She hesitated. We negotiated. She would go, but only to the service; I would drive her over and back; and if she felt sick, she'd call and I'd be over in five minutes to pick her up.

As I buttoned her blouse that evening—her arthritic fingers couldn't easily manipulate the small buttons—I looked at her, in a skirt for the first time in weeks and wearing her wig.

"You look so pretty, Mom," I said.

She beamed.

When the effects of chemotherapy made even the short Friday service more than she could manage, attending the Passover seder, a ceremonial meal held each spring at the temple, became her goal. She accepted the fact that other activities were beyond her now, but the seder, just the seder, she wanted to attend. Passover beckoned like a beloved face in a crowd of strangers, a precious connection with her identity as a Jew while much of the rest of her life was wandering in new and fearsome territory.

Would she be well enough? We fretted over the prospect for weeks and sent in our reservations with crossed fingers. I would go with her, as would her sister-in-law, Evelyn. The evening arrived, and, yes!, she was able.

"Why is this night different from all other nights?" A child has asked this question at Passover for more than a thousand years. That night *was* different for my mother—in an unexpected way. At the end of the meal, she leaned over to me and whispered, "Let's go."

I asked no questions. We got up and rushed out. Mom fainted outside the building. Evelyn helped me get her into the car and accompanied us home. We put Mom to bed and, although she recovered from the episode, she didn't attend temple again while undergoing chemo. The rabbi visited her at home, however, and they talked politics—almost like old times.

Mom supported me, too, in my religious practices, despite the fact that they were unfamiliar to her. I tried to avoid hurting her by not harping on these; yet, avoiding sensitive issues doesn't mean hiding them. I needed to find a middle way. "The middle way," the keynote of Buddhist training—indeed, a synonym for Buddhism—is not a pat formula, for it differs with each situation. Action needs to be rooted in morality; that is invariable. Otherwise, the guideline is broad: behavior should reflect sensitivity and compassion for all involved in the situation at hand. Here, I felt the middle way meant being open and natural about the fact that I was meditating in my room daily.

I waited for a chance. Then, one morning near the beginning, I responded to her good-morning greeting and added self-consciously, "I just finished meditating. I do it every day." The slight tension in my belly eased as I said it. It's interesting how the body reacts when you say what you need to say. Mom's simple, neutral response also helped. "Oh," she replied.

In addition to meditating in my room, I found that I needed a place away from the drama in the house where I could be quite and meditate for a few hours each week. I called a nearby Carmelite monastery and explained my situation to the Mother Superior. She replied, "God brought you to our chapel, and you are welcome here."

A little hesitant, I told Mom about my plans. Maybe she'd become resigned to what she likely viewed as my peculiarities. Maybe a Catholic monastery was more familiar than the Buddhist one I'd been living in, or maybe her disease left her with little extra energy to object. In any case, she replied amiably, "Okay."

"That went down smoothly," I thought, relieved.

A few weeks later, after I'd gone to the chapel three or four times, Mom inquired, "Do you know anyone there?"

"No," I replied.

"Does anyone talk to you?" she asked.

"No. People usually come in, pray, and then leave."

"Do you say hello to anyone?" she tried again.

"Yes!" I affirmed happily. "Once in a while when I'm leaving or taking a break, I say hello to someone."

This wasn't exactly conviviality, but at least it went a step in the direction of meeting her expectations.

I realized that the silence of the chapel, which I loved and which seemed natural to me, was foreign to her. Jewish services were, in my experience, warm social affairs embroidered with comings and goings and, outside, lots of shaking of hands, chatting, children running, parents calling, teenagers flirting. Why should I expect my mother to understand my practice of going alone to a Catholic church and sitting for hours in silence?

She surprised me, though. She may not have understood, but many times when I was leaving for the chapel, she said sweetly, "Have a good time, Honey."

Which was what I was doing.

Shoes and Jeans and Silver Hair and Not-So-Silly Things

"What are you wearing these days?" Marcia asked on the phone. I talked regularly with Marcia, who lived in the Washington, D.C., area. Her question wasn't silly. She knew I'd gotten rid of most of my clothes a year earlier in preparation for becoming a monk. Dresses, skirts, blouses, coats, slacks, shoes—almost all went, as did my car, my apartment, and most of my household possessions.

"Pretty much what I wore at the Abbey," I replied.

I'd bought a couple of dresses since I'd come to St. Louis— I missed dresses—and Mom generously let me wear any of her clothes that fit. Mostly, however, I wore the jeans, khakis, and tee shirts that I'd worn at Shasta Abbey. They were comfortable.

And Birkenstocks. In St. Louis I became sensitive to the habitat of Birkenstocks. Commonly found on the East and West Coasts, they were relatively rare in the Midwest, especially among women my age. I wore these orthopedically designed, inelegant sandals summer and winter—in cold weather I donned heavy socks, as I had in the monastery's cloisters.

"A flower child a few decades late," I thought with a wry inner smile.

I hadn't been a flower child in the 1960s, despite two undergraduate years at Oberlin College, a cradle of flower-childism. As a younger adult, quality clothes (meaning expensive) had been my preference. Now, in my fifties, it was jeans, Birkenstocks, no makeup, and, egads, gray hair.

The gray had appeared in my twenties, and by my late thirties, it was so predominant I tried proactively to staunch the flow of age by coloring my hair. This was a problem because I enjoyed swimming, and the chlorine in pools gave my chemically treated hair a greenish cast. I was embarrassed one day when putting on an army-green dress to notice that the dress and my hair were almost the same hue. So be it. Green hair was less objectionable than not swimming. As for the other alternative—to stop coloring my hair—it wasn't even a consideration.

When I went to the monastery, however, the coloring stopped. Tinting one's hair at a monastery is a ludicrous proposition. Especially at a monastery like Shasta Abbey, where the monks, conforming to Buddhist monastic tradition, shave their heads.

Tinted hair amid a bald group might be ludicrous, but I thought about it wistfully more than once. As the gray began to show, I swung between wishing it would turn quickly and hoping it never would. I felt most comfortable wearing a hat.

Once all of the artificial color had grown out, a process that seemed to take forever, the results were shocking. My hair wasn't gray. It was silver—so bright, it caught me by surprise each time I passed the mirror in the women's bathroom.

Accustomed to dowdy green, I felt conspicuous.

The humor in this little drama was clear to me. So was the value I placed on appearances. In a setting and spiritual practice dedicated to seeing into the ephemeral nature of phenomena, I was stuck on a $5.50 bottle of hair coloring. My mind didn't let go of that bottle or of the yearning for youth its contents indulged. But at least I was aware of my clinging, and the effort to be aware is itself an offering.

Such an offering of awareness is finally a matter of faith. More important than success at any given moment, the willingness to *try* to be aware, to try again and again despite mistakes and lapses, is one of the greatest gestures a person can make. For each offering is an acknowledgement of the truth underlying inner spiritual training. This truth is that awareness leads to clarity, and clarity leads out beyond our notion of selfhood. This is what the ancient Zen master, Dogen, meant when he wrote, "To study Buddhism is to study the self. To study the self is to forget the self. To forget the self is to be enlightened by all things."

My discomfort about my hair turning gray wasn't the first time I'd faced my touchiness about aging. I had found that life offers the same lessons over and over in different guises until we learn them deeply.

I knew what this one was: to learn that age is just age. Aging is a natural process in which no phase is inherently good or bad. Yet, my newly gray hair notwithstanding, I still wanted to hang onto youth, to hoodwink myself and everybody else into believing I was still young.

Learning can be so slow! Real learning, I mean. Not just the ability to write "age is just age" on the blackboard a hundred times, but learning at the molecular level, where I wouldn't wince at the sight of my gray head in the mirror and want to minutely inspect each new facial sag and wrinkle.

Anger or frustration over all this was pointless because it would merely create a further lesson to be learned: the need to let go of anger and frustration. I chose instead to try to accept middle age and my reactions to it with honesty, humor, and hope—the hope that by being mindful of them time and again, I'd someday be free of my hangups about aging. And this tied into an even deeper issue—the inner work I needed to do—which was to bring mindfulness to all the shifty little moments of life.

Mindfulness has a very specific meaning in Buddhist practice. It means being fully attentive to whatever is at hand, without inner comments or judgments or habitual reactions. Moment-by-moment attention is prodigiously difficult, for our minds have a life-long habit of encrusting experience with beliefs, fears, and desires that prevents us from seeing things as they truly are. Training in mindfulness means retraining the mind by catching oneself time and again in unmindful thoughts and deeds and seeing that, for one thing, age is just age.

Since I didn't see it yet, my gray hair ambushed me anew in St. Louis. When Mom first saw my all-gray head, she was kind. "It looks nice," she remarked. But a few days later, she sweetly asked if I planned to color it again. She was hoping I would remarry, and I think she feared that no man would be interested in a gray woman.

74

On the other hand, my Aunt Evelyn, an octogenarian, was enthusiastic. "There's nothing prettier than a young face surrounded by gray hair!" she declared.

Maybe.

In St. Louis, where most women, like most women everywhere, try to look younger than their years, I felt I looked older than mine. Ticket takers at the movies assumed I was a senior. Baggers at the supermarket asked if I needed help carrying my groceries to the car. Me? Who not ten years earlier, when I lived on a farm, regularly handled fifty-pound bags of horse feed and bales of hay three-quarters my size! "Do they ask the same question to women with colored hair?" I wondered.

Perhaps in self-defense, I decided I was on the cusp of a New Age among women. Every so often, I saw a woman in her forties or fifties who had also bowed to nature and was completely gray.

"Very attractive," I thought, not without self-interest.

L iving in St. Louis gave me a chance to wear jewelry again. Although I'd disposed of most of my belongings, I'd kept about ten boxes filled with things I wasn't ready to part with. A box here, a box there, my few possessions were scattered from coast to coast, stored for me by kind friends and relatives. In one I'd sent to Mom for storage was my jewelry.

Bracelets, earrings, and, most happily, I now wore a watch that Dad had given Mom some fifty years earlier and which she, in turn, had given to me. Small and delicate with a rose-gold case set with two small stones and a cord band, the watch, significantly, ran slow. I had to remind myself that it was later than I thought.

There was an appealing incongruity about wearing this watch on my wrist—a lovely piece of jewelry on the arm of one whose feet had almost crossed the monastic threshold. It seemed emblematic of the ambiguous space I lived in. I was neither a monk nor fully not a monk. I inhabited a place in-between, unsure how long I would be here, but deeply glad I was, and uncertain how I would change as a result of life with my dying mother, but knowing I would.

The Bottom Line

The fourth of the month was for Laclede Gas and the Sewer District, the tenth for Union Electric, and the twenty-third for paying her credit card. The automatic social security deposit was recorded on the third.

My mother was well organized. She didn't lose bills on her desk for a week or two, then rush to pay at the last minute. Nor did she take on faith that Visa got it right and give statements a mere once-over to check for egregious errors, instead of verifying receipt by receipt. Those practices were more my style.

From Dad, Mom had inherited financial responsibilities. She was proud of her ability to handle her financial affairs, and, though she seldom discussed them, she clearly was doing a good job.

When Mom was hospitalized, the bill-paying duties fell to me. I assumed, correctly, it turned out, that she wouldn't be able to fully shoulder them again. It seemed important now, when her life was dissolving, for Mom to keep as much control over her affairs as she was able and to have continuity in her routines.

So I organized. One day, before she left the hospital, I told her I needed to consult about the bills. I made an "appointment" with her for a day when no medical tests or other distractions were scheduled. Then I bundled together the unpaid bills, yellow sticky notes, a blank pad of paper, and a pen, putting them into a shopping bag, a gaily flowered pink one, that I carried to the hospital each day in an affirmation of cheeriness.

Before I arrived at the appointed time, shopping bag in hand, I made sure to pay the bills that were due immediately. Slipshod financial housekeeping at the outset would have marred my attempt to promote her peace of mind.

I came away from our meeting—actually, two of them, because she was too weak to do it at one go—with yellow sticky-flags waving from each bill: "pay on the 15th ," "pay—30th," or "call and verify amount." And Mom emerged with a feeling of being in touch with her affairs and the assurance they were being handled as she wished.

Most of all, however, I think she came away with a sense of relief. Although she didn't voice doubts about my ability to pay the bills or manage her filing system, she was impressed—quite excessively, I thought—when I displayed what seemed to me paltry skills that a sixth-grader could master.

Maybe I was oversensitive. I'd been responsibly managing my financial affairs for years, but—truth be told—I'd made a few mistakes in the past. Mothers have long memories. I think I'd gained a reputation with her for having less than a keen interest in financial matters, which was true enough. I attended to them by necessity and will rather than from interest. But I *did* attend to them. Now, when Mom repeatedly expressed pleasure tinged, I detected, with surprise at my efficiency, I commented, a little dryly, "It's not all that hard." Why go after the matter with a club? Why dig up stale issues? Now was now.

By the second month, Mom was back home with the diagnosis of terminal illness. She picked up her office duties again, but even a half-hour's work exhausted her. So I brought the bills and other matters to her in her tall yellow chair, which seemed to dwarf her frail figure but where she was comfortable, and we continued the sticky-note-and-pad-of-paper routine.

Soon, I inherited the job fully. As office manager, I found other administrative matters needed attention, too. Mom wanted to review details of her estate with me. Characteristically, she and Dad, especially Dad, had set up the legal structure with lawyers years earlier, and she hadn't questioned it since.

The more we reviewed, the more *I* questioned, however. Was this the best structure? I didn't know. But it seemed important to find out. Without saying anything to Mom—I didn't want to alarm her—I began to read, talk with knowledgeable people, and listen to advice.

My travels in the world of estate planning soon revealed that there *were* better ways. For one thing, a revocable living trust protects an estate from probate and lawyers' fees. Mom didn't have one. Also, we could save money if I were appointed her personal representative. Years earlier, Dad had arranged for a local bank to perform these administrative duties after her death because Gail and I lived out of town. But now things had changed. Living in St. Louis, I could handle these matters as readily as an institution, and I wouldn't charge the estate to do it.

The issue was delicate. Most of us find major change upsetting, and the upset would likely be greater for Mom, because she was conservative by nature and her declining health made most changes hard to think about. How much harder it would be to consider changes in arrangements fixed by Dad, which held for her nearly the sanctity of law.

My heart beat hard and my adrenaline raced as I considered how to present the suggestions so she wouldn't resist out of hand. I became aware I was edging perilously close to manipulation, and this was a problem.

Manipulation creates bad karma. It means barging into areas where one should not properly be, and there is bound to be some kind of negative effects, even if the immediate goal is attained. Adults need to make their own choices and take responsibility for their actions. My parents had planned the estate with the advice of lawyers, and I knew that if I pushed Mom into making changes against her will, I would be forcing her to forego responsibility in order to accept my view. Taking advantage of her newly won respect for me in financial matters and of her ill health would likely create resentment, a whole crop of it, sprouting like dandelions on a spring lawn. That would devalue both of our lives a bit.

I understood, too, that, on a more intangible level, manipulation leads away from inner freedom. By pressing what I thought to be the best interests of the estate, I risked getting caught in my personal agenda. I could lose sight of the higher interest in the matter, which was Mom's peace of mind, and, through my attachment, get mired in a sticky place. That's not freedom.

Dropping the matter, however, didn't seem right either. Have you ever noticed that the more closely you look at what's going on in your life, the more complicated things seem to become initially? The notion, which at one time I might have held, that "of course I should urge the most expedient action here," wasn't adequate now. Moreover, this complexity wasn't simply an inconvenience to be resented, as I once might have done. Beauty lies right in the thick of complexity, in the texture of it, like a Renaissance painting with all its shades and nuances. Refusing to recognize it would mean opting to live on the simplistic level often portrayed in soap operas and mass circulation magazines. Something deep within knows that's a caricature.

On the other hand, while it is valuable to perceive and savor complexity, there is no need to be overwhelmed by it. The way through lies in mindfulness. If I could be certain that my motives aligned with the best interests of the situation, a course of action would fall into place without serious confusion. Here is where the body offers a gift. For the body is wise; it knows when our motives are in alignment, it knows the bottom line, even when we don't. It tugs at us, though often only subtly, to tell us when we're out of line. Our job is to be sensitive to the signal.

As I thought about changing the structure of my mother's estate, I did feel the tug. It was right there in my solar plexus, warning me, none too softly, "Whoa, don't get righteous!"

So, over and over to make sure: the changes were standard features in estate planning, nothing exotic. They wouldn't alter the terms of Mom's will, but they would protect her intentions. I wasn't advocating them because I alone stood to gain; both Gail and I would equally benefit. I felt certain that had Dad been alive, he would have supported them, for he was a careful planner. And our discussions showed that Mom was unaware of these options. So it seemed possible that even now, at this late hour, her conscientiousness and practicality might induce her to consider changes. It all felt right, a go-ahead, but with the understanding, the agreement with myself, that if Mom objected, I wouldn't try to muscle the matter through.

Searching for a skillful way to present it, I recognized that thoroughness at one blow wouldn't work. I couldn't announce, "Your estate isn't set up well; this is how I think it should be," then proceed to lay out options, point by point. That would be overwhelming, and it would raise Mom's resistance. So I told the truth—that my friend Hal, whom Mom respected, had set up a revocable living trust for his wife, children, and grand-children, and he urged us to look into doing the same; that I knew little about estate planning; and that maybe she and I could explore the matter together.

It worked. She was willing. We did it slowly, over weeks, allowing time for each new spoonful of information to digest. I read her passages from library books I'd borrowed, and we talked about issues. Finally, after we had thought our way into the matter, discussed it thoroughly, and knew our questions, I consulted her lawyer. His "yes" on all counts clinched the matter. We started legal proceedings. By then, Mom had no doubts.

I felt a sense of contentment, even pride, in the outcome. The estate was on sounder grounds, and I had handled the matter skillfully. Further, what might have been traumatic to our relationship—my good intentions notwithstanding—resulted instead in deepened mutual respect. I respected Mom's willingness to undertake these major changes. And, by golly, she respected my role in the matter, though I doubt she grasped the extent of my angst. At least I hope she didn't.

A Mother Lode

"Your mother is a strong woman. And she's well educated—you can see that."

Sitting next to Mom, shoulder to shoulder, on her bed, I repeated what our neighbor had said to me earlier that day. Her jaw dropped, revealing a mouth empty of the dentures that had begun to hurt her gums, the latest targets of her trigger-happy disease. Such praise from Dr. Etienne! My parents had known him cordially for years, and Mom respected him so deeply that now she could barely credit his words. How could anyone of his stature think highly of her? She didn't have to spell out her reaction for me to get a sense of it.

Reaching over, she tilted my head toward her and whispered into my ear, "Do people have to be dying for people to say nice things about them?"

"No, Mom," I assured her. "People have been saying nice things about you for a long time, and Dr. Etienne meant it. He wasn't just being nice."

She smiled a little smile, maybe in disbelief, but I think she was pleased.

My mother's formal education ended after high school. She seldom spoke of it; many of her friends didn't know. Maturing during the Great Depression, she had gone to work after graduation to help support her family because, along with the stock market, the family business had collapsed, for a second time. First was the "pants factory," as Mom called their earlier, men's ready-to-wear venture; then the sausage factory, which, according to family rumor, had been sabotaged by an employee secretly in the pay of a rival from a neighboring state. Just out of high school, Mom got a job. Then Sam Stone became part of her life. She met the young pharmacist at his store, and within six months of their first date, they married. "Not a good idea. Get to know a man better before you make such a commitment," they later counseled Gail and me. It was wise advice, belied, however, by the fact that their marriage was a success.

All of this left my mother with little time for formal education. I don't recall her complaining about inadequacy, but clearly she hungered for more. She was motivated, I think, not by social pressure but because she loved the stuff of it. Yet, shy and of a generation whose women didn't commonly return to school, she was intimidated by the prospect of enrolling in a college-level course. "I'm not sure I could study hard enough. I'm out of practice," she admitted to me once, explaining why, although she'd taken a few adult education courses, she was reluctant to tackle something more demanding.

She did it on her own instead. With the same determination that enabled her to point-blank quit smoking after a thirty-year career in that habit, she got herself an education. A long-time chain reader, Mom always had a book going. She read two papers a day and conversed knowledgeably about current affairs, especially the Washington political scene.

"You would have been a good political activist," I observed a few times.

"Oh, no!" she demurred, for she found distasteful the public attention that even a letter to the editor would bring.

"What about writing a political column?" I teased, waiting for her horrified response—and receiving it.

For years, I took my mother's efforts to educate herself for granted. In fact, I didn't notice. Anymore than I noticed my breath or my heartbeat, for they were too close.

Actually, there was more to it. I've long been ambivalent about my own formal education. I like to think I wear my Ph.D. degree lightly. I seldom refer to it, or even think about it. You don't need a Ph.D. in a monastery or when caring for your mother.

I love learning, and much time and money have gone into the accumulating of it. Toward the end of my undergraduate training, however, a powerful spiritual experience made me recognize the limitations of intellectual attainment. I refused to attend my graduation ceremony that spring, and shortly thereafter, I returned my diploma to the chancellor. In the fervor of my resolve, I told him that my education—I'd been a philosophy major—was meaningless. He was stunned, and my parents, who had footed the considerable bills, were naturally distraught. A week or so later, having reconsidered my action, I went back to the chancellor's office and retrieved the diploma.

It was waiting for me at the secretary's desk—no explanations were needed. I went on to acquire two additional degrees, and, more paradox, I taught part-time at universities, filling the minds of others with the intellectual information about which I was so ambivalent.

My understanding about the limitations of intellectual attainment deepened with time. I recognized that while intellectual information is useful and important, the knowledge that already resides within us is of another and higher order altogether. Usually obscured in the course of life, this innate knowing is accessible to those who seek it. The effort lies not in putting information into the mind, but in becoming quiet enough to begin to hear what's been there all along.

My spiritual work to uncover the Original Mind (one of many terms for the unnamable Knowing within each of us) didn't eliminate the pride, even arrogance, I felt over my intellectual achievement. Although I tried to let go of these unsavory qualities, they kept a tenacious hold, and they were a subtle, unintended part of my manner of relating to my mother.

Without giving it much thought, I assumed I knew many things that she didn't. I remember a conversation about kayaking in which I launched into an explanation of what a kayak was and how it differed from a canoe. Once I completed this neat little discourse, Mom replied quietly, but with an edge, "I know." I didn't have the grace to apologize.

In Buddhism, there are precepts for moral behavior, much as there are in Judaism and Christianity. In fact, the Ten Commandments are exact counterparts in some cases for the Buddhist precepts, though the sense behind them differs. With regard to the Ten Commandments, the understanding is that failure to obey results in Divine punishment. Fear and guilt are means to keep us obedient. On the other hand, the Buddhist precepts are guidelines to enable us to live cleanly, for in that direction lies freedom and happiness for ourselves and others. Failure to observe them will naturally result in suffering. The Dhammapada, an ancient book of Buddhist verses, says:

> *All actions are led by the mind.*
> *Mind is their master; mind is their maker.*
> *Act or speak with a defiled state of mind*
> *and suffering will follow*
> *as a cartwheel follows the foot of an ox.*

The responsibility is our own. We must bear the consequences of our actions, but at any time, we can choose to do better.

> *Act or speak with a pure state of mind,*
> *and happiness will follow*
> *as your shadow follows you without departing.*

Lay Buddhists take five or ten precepts (depending on the tradition), committing themselves to trying to live a moral life. Monastics take more. One of the Zen precepts is "I will try to do my best to refrain from being proud of myself and devaluing others." I knew where I stood on that one. Actually, I didn't consciously think of the precept when I was explaining kayaks or on the countless other occasions when I made assumptions about limitations of my mother's knowledge. I didn't think, "Uh-oh, I'm breaking a precept here." But I had enough moral sensitivity to be bothered by the dynamics of the kayak interchange. The edge in Mom's voice lingered in my mind and kept nudging me until I began to recognize how often I had been condescending. I was being subtly proud of myself and devaluing her.

I began to look more carefully at who she was. One day, I realized with surprise that she had been making a long and arduous effort to educate herself.

I was deeply moved, and I told her so. Her response revealed that I'd struck a mother lode, a focus that had laced her years, though she hadn't said much about it. She beamed and quietly replied, "I've been trying very hard."

"You're doing a really good job, Mom," I beamed back.

One evening a year and a half before Mom died, when she was in the hospital for testing—doctors hadn't yet determined the nature of her illness—we spoke on the phone, I from the monastery.

"Have a good last night in the hospital," I said as we concluded, knowing she'd be released the next day.

She laughed and declared, "A good night in a hospital is an oxymoron."

Two More Years

"I don't want it!" Mom insisted. Her voice rose on the "want it," faintly resembling the surge of a siren's wail. So unlike her.

"I don't want to go down to the hospital and sit in waiting rooms! I've been through enough! Why don't they leave me alone?"

I agreed. Why didn't they leave her alone? There was no cure for her cancer now, so why was Dr. Anderson urging radiation for one tumor, just one of many? It didn't make sense.

Mom had grown lumpy. Tumors were appearing all over her body, and they were growing at an alarming rate. Most noticeable was the one in the middle of her forehead. Bigger and bigger it got. Like an obscene gesture or a slash of screaming paint across a nuanced canvas, it was an alien presence in our midst.

I tried, but I never fully accepted her disease as a natural part of life, as natural as health and merely its opposite, as dying is the opposite of living.

That is what the master in a Zen story was pointing to when he asked a student how he was. The student replied,

"Fine." The master commented, "That's good."

Soon after, the master asked the same question, and the student, who was struggling with new problems, replied, "Not well." The master commented, "That's good."

His remark wasn't callous or uncaring. The master was pointing to That Which Is Eternal, that which exists within all things, in all conditions and is itself without conditions. The Unconditioned existed in Mom's cancerous tumors as well as in her former relatively good health. Sun-faced Buddha, moon-faced Buddha.

Mom probably didn't live at this profound level of acceptance, but she certainly accepted at some level. She knew that it was pointless to resist her disease and that the time for fighting was past.

And also the time for questioning. Mom seldom asked questions, especially of doctors. For her, doctors held a position close to God and one of greater immediate practicality. And now, she was too sick and too intimately involved to think clearly. When they discussed her treatment, she listened silently, her eyes round and blank. Did those blank eyes reflect respect for the speaker, or did they mask terror at her condition, an unacknowledged terror, perhaps, that made her shut out what was fearful? Maybe she would have been just as happy not knowing.

Her silence left me with the responsibility of trying to understand and explaining to her later on. I'd already learned the importance of these duties. A year earlier, during our first meeting with the oncologist, Mom had heard him say that she was too old to fight for her life, and that it was pointless to undergo chemotherapy. She had been ready to give up. In contrast, I had heard that, with treatment, she would have a fifty-percent chance at survival. Explaining to her my understanding of what the doctor had said had helped her decide to opt for chemo.

Now, I realized that I needed to become my mother's advocate to ensure that she got the best treatment possible, consistent with her own wishes. To begin with, that meant asking questions when she did not, and asking them skillfully. Approaching matters skillfully, called "skillful means" in Buddhism, involves sensitively responding to a situation. The aim is not only to be effective but also to leaven action with morality and compassion. This can be a tall order because it often requires us to refrain from customary responses and to search for the most appropriate ones. These may lie in unfamiliar areas, and they may require that we set aside our personal preferences.

Skillful means is a relief, however. By providing guidelines to action, it cuts through the mental thrashing about that we easily get caught in when we weigh this and that option against our agendas and preferences. The use of skillful means is essentially a spiritual act, for it requires us to momentarily offer up the self.

What skillful means required of me now was to set aside my pride and ask questions when I didn't understand what the doctors were saying. I needed to persist until I received answers I fully understood, even at the risk of appearing dumb. I decided to make question-asking something of an art form. I learned to formulate my questions beforehand, writing them down so that I wouldn't forget during the fast, few minutes of conversation with the doctor. On the many occasions when a doctor's initial explanation baffled me, I tried not to swing toward frustrated antagonism—neither an intimidated "oh, okay" nor a comment like "I don't understand a word you said. Why don't you talk plain English?" Skillful means is finding a middle way.

Once Mom was a hospice patient, our nurse Barbara became our main source of medical information, and, happily, she did speak plain English. But I couldn't expect Barbara to know about the latest treatments for bone pain.

Now that a cure wasn't an option, our goal was to enable Mom to die as comfortably as possible. Her pain, which was sometimes savage, was only a fraction of what could happen later. Wanting to know the range of options available to us, I began to research information about treatments to alleviate cancer-related bone pain.

Friends kindly provided me with information from the Internet. From a friend who worked in oncology research, I learned about a treatment, administered through shots, which if given early enough can forestall certain kinds of cancer pain in the bones. I learned too about a medication newly approved by the FDA that might be helpful. Information led to more information.

Mom was unenthusiastic about my research. When I tried to discuss my findings, she was unresponsive. Her round, blank eyes should have been my clue. Finally, her repeated lack of interest and her several versions, in response to my efforts, of "Dr. Anderson doesn't recommend that," showed me it was pointless to discuss it with her.

What I probably knew vaguely all along became clear to me. I was doing this research as much for my sake as for hers. It comforted me to know the options. It was the difference between walking a path in daylight and stumbling along at night. Caregivers need to take care of themselves, too! Besides, Mom's faith in the medical profession notwithstanding, maybe there *was* something Dr. Anderson had overlooked.

R adiation had never been an option in treating Mom's cancer. When I learned about strontium-89, an advanced treatment for cancer pain, I wanted to explore the advisability of administering it to Mom. I broached the subject with Dr. Anderson and was puzzled when he responded by talking instead about radiating the tumor on Mom's forehead.

He had ruled out other alternatives I'd raised earlier, and he usually patiently explained why. On this occasion, however, his advice was obscure. Aside from the fact that his response seemed a non sequitur, our focus in Mom's care had been pain management, and the tumor on her forehead didn't hurt. Nor was the cosmetic effect a factor. The disfigurement didn't bother her much. No one was looking except her and me, a few family visitors, and hospice support people. Eliminating that one tumor would be like removing one leaf from a lawn strewn with fall leaves and abundant with trees still dropping them.

Barbara, with whom Mom and I discussed the dilemma, provided no clarification. In fact, she made it worse because she checked and found that hospice wouldn't consider the treatment palliative, which is the only kind of care permissible under their mandate. Mom would have to drop out of the hospice program to receive radiation. Though she could re-enroll after the treatment was over, the emotional upset of leaving the protective embrace of hospice made the prospect of radiation even more unappealing. We would be cast out on our own.

Dr. Anderson persisted, though. He even brought a radiologist into the discussion. At first, I thought the radiologist was there to discuss strontium-89 because he would be the one to administer it. But when the receptionist from his office, who'd practically strong-armed us into setting up an appointment, called again to instruct us to bring along x-rays of Mom's skull, I sensed something was fishy. Skull x-rays shouldn't be necessary if Mom were merely getting shots of strontium-89.

That is how my mother came to say "no" to a doctor's advice, maybe for the first time in her life. Her distress was contagious, and I called back and cancelled the appointment. When the receptionist later admitted that the purpose had been to assess the advisability of radiation, we felt indignant. They were trying to hoodwink us for reasons we didn't understand.

"Okay," I thought, "maybe my skillful means haven't been too skillful. I need to find out what's really going on."

In the next conversation with Dr. Anderson, what needed saying finally got said, and it was horrifying. Without radiation, the tumor on her forehead, which now was a half-dollar-sized lump, might grow through her skull and into her brain, causing brain damage and severe pain.

My stomach went queasy. We were prepared for Mom's declining health, but not for brain damage. As though the brain weren't part of the body, we had never considered the possibility of the cancer corroding her bright mind. Hanging up the phone, I paused for a minute to try to quiet my insides. Then, I told Mom.

Suddenly, leaving hospice didn't seem an obstacle. We wanted to know how soon radiation could start. Tomorrow? The day after? We'd already wasted two weeks or more going back and forth between doctors.

As the radiation treatments progressed, the tumor on her forehead slowly disappeared. Mom and I marveled over the transformation, and we were deeply relieved at the danger we had averted. The disease would not invade her mind— at least not as a result of this tumor.

After the last treatment, we sat in an examination room talking quietly, waiting for a final consultation with the radiologist. A kind man with a national reputation, he resembled a small teddy bear. Mom and I had liked him right away. He came into the room to inspect his handiwork. Holding Mom's chin in his hand, he squinted at her forehead appreciatively and said, "You could live another two years."

It was meant as good news, but his comment had the effect of an electric shock. Mom jerked her head toward me and mouthed (she didn't want him to hear), "God forbid!"

He must have noticed, because he turned away as if to give her privacy. Still looking at me, she said it again, this time in a forceful whisper, anguish all over her face, "God forbid!"

In traditional Chinese and Japanese art, nature is not a backdrop against which human lives are centerpieces, as it often is in Western art. In Eastern painting, people are depicted as part of nature—tiny figures seen from behind, walking away from a rowboat, or crossing a little bridge in the lower part of the third panel of a four-panel landscape, or seated in small groups, features indistinct, chatting beneath a pine in a gnarly forest on the side of a mountain that is one of a range of mountains whose bases fade softly into mist at the horizon.

Landscape isn't the centerpiece in these paintings, either. Space is. Space surrounds all, defines all, wraps everything in termless depth. Such paintings are mandalas of sorts. They can be seen to represent the practice of meditation itself. For in meditation we learn to center our awareness in the space surrounding the objects of our lives, which is to say in the space surrounding our body sensations, feelings, emotions, and thoughts. All our lives we identify with these things, thinking we are they, and they continually jerk us about like yo-yos on a string. As we learn to identify from the space between, we now and then glimpse a deeper truth. We begin to realize that we are not what we had previously assumed. We are something less. And something unutterably greater.

When the radiologist spoke and Mom whispered, my meditation training may as well have never happened. Mom and I occupied the center of my landscape, and there was no space—only an opaque vista crammed with dread. Two more years.

I tried to imagine Mom living two more years under the weight of her disease. Even without the tumor on her forehead, it was a horrific prospect. I didn't want her to die, but life burdened by her cancer seemed worse. And I tried to imagine my life during the next two years, but I couldn't do it.

Neither Mom nor I talked much on the way home. When we got there, we did the most sensible thing, not a meditator's way, but one that sometimes feels like the only way when stress seems too great to bear—we went to sleep.

Breaking New Ground

During the period when Mom was undergoing radiation treatments, we spent many hours in the radiologist's waiting room. One day, after settling into our chairs, we looked at the nearby aquarium and wondered, "Where's the little blue fish?" Its fellow inmates—the large electric blue, the flat purple, the orange with a fantail, the yellow pancake and the pink-and-blue striped—dived and darted in their close watery world, somehow managing not to bump into each other. But no little blue. We hoped it hadn't died since our last visit.

"There it is, resting between the rocks," Mom pointed. Relieved, we turned to our reading. I opened a book of poetry, and she picked up *Time* magazine.

We read and we read, which is the way of waiting rooms, and the week's news began to pall. Putting down the magazine, Mom gazed at the fishy dance, performed now by the full company. Then she looked around restlessly.

"Would you like me to read you some of this poetry?" I ventured, thinking it might fill the gap. She moved closer, cocked her head toward me, and prepared to listen.

That was the beginning. In addition to fish watching,

poetry reading became part of our waiting room routine. A radiologist's office is as good a place as any to take the first steps toward an appreciation of poetry!

The road to poetry had its bumps, however. Often after I read a poem, Mom declared, "I don't get it." Her literal mind balked like a horse being asked to wade through a stream for the first time.

"Don't try to make sense of it," I counseled. "Just let it flow over you like water. Enjoy what you enjoy. Don't worry about the rest."

Slowly the music of the language struck a resonance. Elizabeth Bishop became a favorite. One of the first poems I read to her was, appropriately, Bishop's "In the Waiting Room," a poem about an experience a young Elizabeth had as a six-year-old in a dentist's waiting room. It begins:

> *I went with Aunt Consuelo*
> *to keep her dentist's appointment*
> *and sat and waited for her*
> *in the dentist's waiting room. . . .*
> *My aunt was inside*
> *what seemed like a long time*
> *and while I waited I read*
> *the* National Geographic. . .
> *Suddenly, from inside,*
> *Came an* oh! *of pain*
> *—Aunt Consuelo's voice—*
> *not very loud or long.*
> *I wasn't at all surprised. . . .*
> *I might have been embarrassed,*
> *But wasn't. What took me*
> *Completely by surprise*

> *Was that it was* me:
> *My voice, in my mouth.*
> *Without thinking at all*
> *I was my foolish aunt,*
> *I—we—we falling, falling,*
> *Our eyes glued to the cover*
> *of the* National Geographic,
> February, 1918.

Mom's *most* favorite poet, however, was me. She wanted to hear every poem I ever wrote. She liked them all, and she even liked hearing them more than once.

"Oh, yes," she nodded knowingly when I reread a poem some months later, "that's the one you wrote last winter."

She was proud to be privy to its history. What poet doesn't like an appreciative audience, even one that overrates the poems!

I was careful about what I read to her, however. Some I wasn't ready to share. Others, about her illness, might be upsetting. And many, my earlier poems, weren't readily available, being stored in a box somewhere by a friend or relative, along with my other remaining possessions.

When my output of "pleasant" poems ran thin, I decided to try something tougher. I prefaced this poem with the assurance that I'd stop if she found it depressing.

Robin at the Window

For days a robin perches at the window.
Minutes at a time, it faces
the wrong way—in, not out.
Why are you here, little bird?
Indian tales about messengers

from the spirit world don't happen
on a suburban window ledge.

My mother and I watch a film
about the Kalahari.
Desert rains stopped early,
stranding fledgling pelicans
too young to escape with their parents.
Sweltering. One by one,
then in group, they start
to walk the flat, cracked land
that was their lake, their paradise.
Little bodies drop
and no one is there to help.

My mother rises from her chair,
its headrest worn with sweet use.
She squeezes my arm, then walks
to the kitchen to take another Demerol.
Roaring into a new part of her body,
the disease is an engine
that will not be stopped.

I look at the window again.
It's empty now,
but on the panes in robin code,
swipes and flecks of mud
where feather and beak tried hard
to get inside.

Mom liked it. With a faith that only a mother can har-
bor, she assumed my poetry would someday be published. She
asked me to dedicate my first book of poems to her. It was one
of the easiest promises I ever made. I knew the chance of pub-
lication existed somewhere between Timbuktu and the near-
est quasar, but I was moved by her request.

One morning as I walked into the sitting room where Mom had taken her position for the day, she said from her yellow recliner, "I want to read you something I've written."

Her words wriggled like puppies with excitement—her first poem! Taken by surprise, I was touched by her enthusiasm. At a time when depression would have been understandable, she was struggling with a new art form. She was reaching beyond her habitual thought patterns, to express herself in a new way. That's hard at any age!

"I like it," I responded.

"Do you really? That means a lot to me!"

During the next weeks Mom wrote other poems and eagerly read each aloud. One morning, again from her yellow chair, she announced, "I want to ask you something. You keep saying you like my poems, but you don't say anything else. I don't want nice words. I want *real* criticism. Like the kind of things you talk about in poetry classes."

Okay. I breathed deeply and started—lightly, a little at a time and positively. Referring to one of her poems, I said, "The idea here is nice, but 'dark green' probably isn't the most interesting way to describe leaves. How can you say it more vividly?" To illustrate the power of description, I read to her from some of my favorite poets. For a few weeks, until she grew too feeble to continue, we talked about adjectives and line breaks and revision and the fact that good poetry isn't just about pretty things, but about real things. And we read poetry.

"Where've you been all these years? I never knew this before. And I was satisfied with just my newspapers and my books," she declared. "You're the only one who could have taught me this, and I really need it now. Thank you *so* much."

Mom worked hardest on a poem about the trees in her yard. She wrote how she'd planted many of them years earlier and how she'd watched them grow. She wrote about her feeling of loss when one died. And she likened the loss to an echo of another, deeper grief: "I feel a tug at my heart as when I lost my love."

Because her feeble script and her many revisions made the final version of the poem hard to read, I typed it. Our plan was for me to type all of her poems, so we could have a clean copy. But soon, as she grew sicker, her interest shifted from poetry, and I stopped typing.

A few weeks before her death, a storm felled one of her beloved trees. I felt a tug at my heart. The tree skeleton lay in the yard for days, being too heavy for me to move. Under the circumstances, it wasn't a priority anyway.

Waking from a long period of semiconsciousness one afternoon a few days later, Mom asked, "Did a tree fall in the yard?"

"How did you know?" I asked in amazement. "I wasn't going to tell you because I didn't want to bother you!"

Bedbound, she couldn't see the tree from her window and, being a bit hard of hearing, she was less likely to have heard it fall than I. And I hadn't heard it.

In a response that any poet would understand, this literal-minded woman replied, "I don't know how. I just know."

I had written the following poem in the spring of 1996 when my mother was undergoing chemotherapy.

Pansies

Spring is struggling this year,
jousting freezing temperatures
long after the calendar mandates moderation.
Daffodils do battle at roadside;
single-minded, they face down the wind.
Driving back from her chemotherapy,
Mom and I consider pansies,
pansies for the terracotta bowl
on the patio table. Pastel words
flutter in pennants from our lips;
petals adorn our space.
I think of Ai's poems about cruelty.
In her fierce landscape—
all blood and coal and ice—
my words and Mom's would shrivel.
Her poems suddenly loom as tribunal,
charging inanity. I brace,
then breathe: We each choose the colors
of our lives. Loving Mom now, here,
is my artwork, and I'm using pastels,
her picked palette.

Maybe we'll see a movie this afternoon,
a comedy, if she's not too tired.

The "artwork" of my life with Mom had opened dimensions far beyond what I imagined when I wrote those words.

Passover at Last

She made the gefilte fish. Not from scratch, but she specified the brand, the kind of fish, the packing broth, and how many pieces I should buy. Then, the day before the seder, Mom added her special touch. To the ground and boiled fish pieces that resembled fat sausages, she added paprika and other herbs. She baked them under cover at 350 degrees for twenty minutes, then cooled and refrigerated them for a nutty, fuller flavor.

That spring, the Passover seder was going to be at home because Mom was too frail to go to temple. Far from being depressed by the prospect, she was excited. She didn't say so, but later, after she had died, it occurred to me that this was the first seder that she had conducted.

When I was a child, the Passover Eve service celebrating the ancient deliverance of the Jewish people from Egypt was held at the home of Baba and Zaida, Mom's parents. It was a large family gathering, with several of her five brothers and sisters and their spouses and children present. We recited the story, as have Jews for thousands of years, about how the Lord passed over the houses of the Israelites enslaved in Egypt, sparing them, but smiting their enemies; how God delivered them from slavery; how He sustained them in the desert for forty years and then led them to the Promised Land. But, most of all, I remember how we all drank tea from glasses, even the kids, through sugar cubes held in our teeth, Russian style. I liked the way the cubes crumbled in the liquid and the gritty feel as I rolled the crumbles with my tongue against the roof of my mouth until, sweetly, they dissolved.

After Baba and Zaida died, the seder was held at the home of one of Mom's older sisters, where we skipped tea-with-cubes. Later, when Gail and I were adults and had moved away, Dad and Mom held the seders at their home, and Dad conducted the service. And after that, as a widow, Mom celebrated Passover at her temple or with out-of-town relatives.

Now, at last, she would conduct the service herself. For this one night, she would join her father, her husband, and her ancestors back beyond recall, and become chief bearer of this tradition so dear to her.

This time, it would be a quiet affair. Evelyn and Sherry were coming—Mom's sister-in-law and niece. There would be no kids squirming in their chairs or falling asleep on the couch or in beds in other rooms as the meal dragged on. No husbands or sisters or brothers, either.

Beforehand, Mom and I discussed how to set the table in the dining room, a room we now used only on special occasions, which this was.

"Let's do it right," I urged, knowing this would be the last time. "Let's use the silver and the Billingsley Rose."

Because Mom tired easily and none of us were big eaters,

we cut down on all aspects of the service—the ceremonial and the gastronomic. A mini-seder it was to be. Not the four obligatory cups of wine, but one, with refills if anyone wanted, and grape juice as an alternative, because Evelyn didn't drink wine. A stack of matzos—you can't have a seder without matzos, the bland, unleavened bread the ancient Hebrews made in their hasty flight from Egypt. Parsley, as a token of gratitude; an egg, as a free-will offering; and for the bitterness of slavery, horseradish. Under Mom's supervision, I mixed chopped apples, nuts, and raisins and doused them in wine with a pinch of cinnamon for the *haroses,* representing the clay the Israelites used to make bricks in bondage. Roasted lamb shank was out, though—we didn't eat lamb. For the meal itself, departing from tradition, I made chicken *à l'orange* and a wild-and-brown-rice pilaf, small portions of each.

Mom took the lead as we discussed the prayers we'd include in the service. On two crib sheets, one for each of us, we marked her selections from the Haggadah, a book of ancient lineage, copies of which her temple had kindly lent us. We marked who would recite each, for Mom wanted the service to flow without flaw when the time came.

Evelyn and Sherry were appreciative. They said so over and over. "Oh, Blanche, I didn't know you could read Hebrew! You read so well!" Evelyn exclaimed as Mom read from the Haggadah, which is partly in English and partly in Hebrew.

Mom acknowledged the praise nonchalantly, as if it were an everyday accomplishment, but you could see she was pleased. She blossomed in her new role like a daylily on its day.

Which may be why she was keen for me to take photographs.

At just about this time, Mom began to object to having her picture taken. Her face had grown colorless and haggard, and tumors were visible on her bones. But for this occasion, this memorable occasion, she wanted photos. I bought a roll with thirty-six shots, more than enough to do the job.

Before the event I photographed the festive table, with its silver flatware, good china, and, in the center, polished for the ceremony, a silver wine cup for the Prophet Elijah. According to tradition, Elijah enters during the seder and drinks his wine. Kids who are awake enough watch the cup. And if you watch closely, you'll almost see the wine line against the side of the cup grow slightly, ever so slightly, less full, as though someone with an invisible straw were taking the tiniest sip. Then, you'll almost feel his presence.

For our seder, we dispensed with the opening of the door to let Elijah in—that's a kid's job. Besides, if he had a mind to do it, wouldn't he pass right through the door? We didn't open the door, but we did joke about the wine in Elijah's cup, which this time definitely did not go down. I know. I watched.

Elijah's-cup jokes must be among the oldest, most well-worn jokes in history. Centuries of kids and adults were linked to us in those moments by our Elijah's-cup jokes. Not to mention by the more solemn aspects of the service. And isn't that a function of rituals? Solemn or light, they connect us, give us a sense of identity, a place in history. They make the past present.

As I listened to Mom read in Hebrew, I knew that beyond the beauty of our service, beyond its socioreligious functions, in its inner meaning, where all rituals are deeply equivalent, the ceremony itself was not what was most meaningful. The mind we brought to it was. If we could celebrate it with the mind of meditation, which *is* reverence—not necessarily the feeling of reverence but a clear awareness in which reverence resides— then wouldn't we fulfill the ceremony's deepest purpose? Maybe then, we would approach the inner meaning of deliverance to the Promised Land.

This, of course, is an understanding influenced by my Buddhist training. It's the understanding that I brought to the seder that evening, and it's what I tried to be open to as we celebrated.

I don't know if any of us experienced inner deliverance, but we all savored the occasion thoroughly. I photographed Mom and Sherry and Evelyn from different angles; then Sherry took pictures so I could be in them—sitting at my place at the table, standing by Mom, by Evelyn, by both.

A few days later, I finished the roll by snapping pictures of the pansies in the garden. Then, as I stood at the kitchen counter, camera in hand and Mom beside me, a moment's lapse. Letting impatience and my natural ineptitude with things mechanical get the better of my sense of discipline, I flipped open the camera lid without rewinding, and I exposed the film.

Mom was disappointed. So was I.

"I'm really sorry, Mom. Really sorry," I repeated.

Generously she replied, "Well, we all make mistakes. We can have another meal soon with Sherry and Evelyn, and you can take new pictures."

"Yes, let's do that," I agreed.

But I think we both knew it wouldn't happen, and it didn't.

Symbols and Beyond

In the dappled light of a spring afternoon, when occasions when Mom would still be well enough to venture out could be counted on your fingers, she and I stood arm in arm before my father's grave, the burial site of her dear Stoney. We both knew our next visit to this spot would be at her funeral.

Her gravesite was alongside Dad's, adjoining plots crowned with a double granite tombstone. His side was inscribed with his name, birth and death dates, a prayer in Hebrew commending his soul to eternal life, and a commemoration— "Loving and beloved husband and father." The other half, at the head of Mom's plot, was waiting for her. No question who would be lying there some day. The tombstone said it: Blanche Olschansky Stone. Except for the date of her death and the commemoration, the inscription was already complete.

Perhaps it was merely the monument company's policy, when selling a double tombstone, to do two for one and to put the finishing touches on later, but it had profound implications for Mom's view of her future. It was a commitment to remain Blanche Olschansky Stone, Sam Stone's wife, to the end of her days.

I asked her once, a few years after Dad had died, if she'd consider remarrying. She replied, "Oh, no, I don't want to spend the rest of my life taking care of some old man."

Which said to me that she *had* thought about it and had rejected the idea. It was a practical response, but a partial one. She didn't need to say the rest. The fact that she still spoke in the plural—"our house," "our bedroom"—said it for her.

"Still," I thought, standing by the grave, "it's a little morbid, this looking at a stone that will proclaim your existence long after it's past." The headstone comforted her, though, and that was the important thing.

Visiting Dad's grave was a pilgrimage, one Mom and I made periodically. But only on sunny, warm days—Mom found visits in gloomy weather depressing. Today, as on other occasions, we brought a carnation to tuck into the periwinkle covering the grave. Anything more ostentatious would be removed by the caretaker. It was cemetery policy.

Ever since Dad had died twelve years earlier, Mom had been bringing red carnations to his grave, but today's flower was pink. She handed it to me, and I threaded the stem through the matted bedding to prevent the flower from being blown by wind. The blossom glimmered against the dark leaves.

Eyeing its pinkness, I thought, "It's fitting. Today's flower is different because today is different—it's her last time."

Mom, with her literal turn of mind, likely accepted that the flower was pink because the florist had run out of red ones. Period. For me, however, the color change was symbolic. Why today of all days had the florist run out of red ones?

My mind delights in symbolism. I revel in it, looking for

hidden meanings. I find that symbols invest events with wonder. They are an affirmation, within the ordinary, of something greater than the ordinary, a connection with Mystery.

The art of symbology can get out of hand, however. You read meaning into an event and detect symbols that confirm your interpretation, but later discover you were wrong. Then what? Do you reinterpret the event? How many times do you do that and find that you were wrong before you give up? And what about negative symbols, those you don't want? You write a letter to a lover from whom you haven't heard in a suspiciously long time; then you spill coffee on it, or drop it in the mud on the way to the post office, or dream he's been unfaithful. The symbolic message is clear, and you grieve before you receive his response. You may even redraft the letter, giving it a new whiny tone that reflects your premonition. Of course, the tone may then prompt just the response you fear.

We need to see things as they are, without adding our meanings to them. Experiencing the reality that resides within the bald moment means experiencing Mystery directly, not just thinking about it and wishing for it. From this perspective, the Mystery that I and other wonderseekers find in symbols becomes a symbol itself, for it is once removed from the actual experiencing of it.

Yet, as a long-time symbologist, I have found it hard to drop the practice. My mind bolts toward interpretation, even while I'm cautioning myself against its hazards. I've never been able to ignore the fact that sometimes the juxtaposition of events *is* extraordinary. Such things always make me catch my breath and bow in wonder. I've finally learned, however, to acknowledge a symbol (or what I think is one) and let it pass. I try not to let it dominate my thoughts and emotions, and I certainly try not to act on it right away. Whether the symbolism appears to be auspicious or depressing, I try to greet it with a degree of equanimity and continue on my way.

More recently, I've come to allow for the possibility of a natural explanation for at least some seemingly wondrous events. It's an explanation that fits right into Buddhist observations about cause and effect. Because our thoughts are a subtle form of energy, maybe, under some circumstances, thoughts have the power to manifest concretely in ways that are beyond our consciousness. Our thoughts are intention, and maybe some of the synchronous effects that we observe are simply natural consequences.

In any case, as Mom and I stood at the foot of the grave, now adorned with the pink carnation, my attention turned to her. I squeezed her arm, and she responded, squeezing mine. We were solemn but not teary. After a few moments of silence, Mom commented, "The periwinkle needs trimming." We bent down, plucked a few weeds and tucked straying stems back into the bed.

As we prepared to leave the gravesite, I glanced around and asked, "Where's Jack? I don't see him."

During our other visits, Jack, the septuagenarian caretaker, had come over and companionably chatted with us as we slowly walked back to the car. "Whose people are you?" he had wanted to know the first time we'd met. He meant which grave did we belong to. We each have our perspectives on life. When we told him, he announced, "I know the grave. I know all the graves here." He said it proudly, as though claiming familiarity with landmarks in Paris. He'd been caretaking there for years.

We had a lengthy conversation that first time. Ever since I'd read Hamlet in a high school English class, I held a notion that grave diggers and, by extension, anyone else working in a cemetery, had a special wisdom that set them apart from ordinary folks. At a break in the conversation, I asked sweetly, "Do any of the people buried here ever talk to you?" I was careful not to say "ghosts" or "spirits." I didn't want him to think I was weird.

"Hell, no!" he replied. "My wife is buried here and even she doesn't talk to me!"

This wasn't the response I'd been anticipating. It didn't square at all with my sentimental, high school notions. As we left, Mom, who evidently was unburdened by illusions in this respect, observed simply, "That man has been working in the cemetery too long. He's lonely."

Jack came over to talk each time we finished our gravesite visit. We learned that at seventy-eight, he wanted to retire. "I've been in this business too long," he declared. "I'm bored." He confided that he was looking for a nice eighteen-year-old girl who could cook. Marriage and a cruise were also on his agenda. Turning to me during one conversation, he asked, "Do you cook?"

"Yes," I replied. "But I'm not eighteen," I hastily added, in case this was an off-handed proposal.

"Oh."

During our last visit to the cemetery, Jack's absence, like the pink carnation, struck me as unusual. I was prepared to see cosmic significance in the fact that on this, Mom's last visit to the gravesite, our customary companion was absent.

In response to my query about Jack's whereabouts, Mom commented, "Maybe he retired." Straightforward, sensible, without an emotional overlay. Had she secretly studied Buddhism?

We wondered if Jack had found his eighteen-year-old. But not for long. As we drove away, our attention shifted to an errand we needed to run before going home and to a complex intersection en route, one I wasn't familiar with.

"Left," Mom pointed. Her index finger, which was crooked, pointed right. With two choices for the turn, I hesitated halfway across. The light changed, and an onslaught of cars came at us from several directions. There was no choice except to push through. Mom helped with the effort.

"Excuse us, excuse us," she sang to cars as we forged on.

Navigating the intersection, I wondered if a policeman were going to arrest me for running a red light. While keeping my eyes focused on traffic, not looking around for police, I formulated my response. I would try to enlist his sympathy. I told Mom, "If a policeman stops us, I'll explain that I'm on my way back from visiting my father's grave."

Picking up on the unspoken rationale behind my statement, she volunteered, "And I'll tell him I'm a hospice patient."

I didn't have to search for cosmic significance in her words. The meaning was clear: it was the meaning of love. More responsive to my silent intent than to the gravity of her own situation, her comment was so poignant that I felt I couldn't breathe on it lest it shatter.

What's in a Name?

It was a lie. Whatever else it signified, my "I'm on my way back from visiting my father's grave," as I dodged traffic with the light against me, was a line geared to manipulate a policeman's response. It seemed justified at the time—in fact, I didn't question it—but it wasn't true. I wasn't running the red light because I was too upset to think straight, as my comment implied. I was running it because I was unsure of my directions and had gotten stuck in the middle. Maybe this sounds like a trivial difference, but it isn't really, when you consider the motivation behind it.

And the imaginary dialogue with a policeman was just part of the story. There was also the matter of the name I tried to give my mother.

I've always found multiple names for beings close to me. The animals I've lived with, judging by a name tally, could have almost made a zoo. Cats, dogs, horses—each responded to all of his or her names. I wasn't searching for that quintessential name that poet Pablo Neruda had in mind when he asked, "What was the name of that cat?" That's the name known only in silence. No, these names flowed abundantly, part of my ongoing conversations with animals.

With my mother, however, it was different. I had never used most of the standard forms of address—not "Mother," an appellation in which, as a young adult, I'd found an appealing dignity, or "Mamma" or "Ma" or, as is fairly common these days, her first name, "Blanche." To me, she was "Mom," just "Mom." At the end when I lived with her, however, things changed. Then, names came without effort, playfully—"Moms," "Mums," "Mommykins."

Our relationship naturally expressed in mother-daughter terms, changing subtly with time. When I became her caregiver, Mom occasionally called me "Mom." Then, we'd laugh and brush past her "mistake." From her point of view, I was Daughter and she was Mother, and what you called Mother was "Mom." The new names that I added toward the end were loving variations, and she welcomed them.

Many years before, when I was in my early twenties, a shocking day came when I realized that my parents were human beings. Like most children, I hadn't been able to see past the Mommy-Daddy-childness of the relationship. Suddenly, without consciously having sought it, a new perspective clobbered me into recognizing that my parents had an identity apart from their relationship to me. With strengths and weaknesses, interests and aversions, loves and fears, my parents, like all people, were shaped by their experiences and were trying to do a good job at their lives as they understood it. They succeeded and failed, they were vulnerable, and their vulnerability was achingly precious. I couldn't articulate these insights at the start, but I felt them with an intensity that was nearly paralyzing.

The new view seemed surreal, like when you look outside during a solar eclipse—nothing has changed but everything has. I couldn't return to the old familiarity, though I tried. I wanted to. Having been thrust into alien territory, I had no choice but to learn to live there. Much later I understood that the shift had freed me to become an adult. It enabled me to relate to my parents, not only as a daughter, but also from a less conditioned place, as one being who was trying to connect with two others.

Now, as I lived with Mom amid the flush of her new names, an idea formed. Could I help her receive the same gift I'd been given when I was jolted into seeing her and Dad on their own terms? If I joggled her a little, could I help her see me, even for an instant, as a person, rather than primarily as a daughter?

"A good friend. Why can't we sometimes be friends who happen to be mother and daughter?" I thought longingly. "Of course, the odds are against it; she's reaching for certainties now, not for new vistas, especially not one that tinkers with our relationship. Still . . . "

These thoughts slowly took shape around "Blancheykins." "Blancheykins"—I chose it carefully. It was friendlier than "Blanche." You can't say it without a smile in your voice. It wouldn't plunge her into the Arctic; the name was a jaunt to a summer beach, the kind of name a dear friend might use, but not her daughter.

It was a big job for one name to do. I knew that. Undeterred by common sense, not to mention by compassion, I got set to play God. Or, at least, to be an experimentalist. I got set to snap Mom out of her sense of the familiar and to make her my unsuspecting subject. Overlooked in my zeal was the fact that we already *were* friends, and that I was cutting matters rather finely by quibbling with her habit of placing her maternal role before friendship.

"Your turn, Blancheykins," I laughed as I inaugurated the name during a game of UpWords, at a point when she was doing very well. I planned to use it only in reassuring circumstances.

She paused; then she made her move.

Each time I used the name in the following days, I felt her inner pause while she tried it on for size. Finally, several "Blancheykinses" later, she decided it didn't fit.

"I don't like that name. Please don't use it again," she said quietly one day.

I didn't insist. All that laundry folding *had* taught me something. Besides, I knew how objectionable it is to be called a name you don't like. At present, it doesn't matter much what I'm called, as long as it's said with kindness. When I was young, however, at the time the new view of my parents rocked my life like an earthquake, I also outgrew my name. "Susie" was fine for a girl, but suddenly I found I was no longer comfortable with it. Mom and Dad did their best to comply when I asked them to call me "Susan," though they often ended up calling me "Honey" or "Suz" instead. So now, when Mom asked me not to address her as "Blancheykins," she didn't have to ask twice. After that, "Mommykins" became one of my favorite names for her. She liked "Mommykins."

Months later, as I began to write this, I was surprised to hear an unlovely theme. Moreover, I noticed that the same theme resonated in the comment I'd concocted for the policeman—the manipulation theme. In both cases, although it hadn't been my intention, my words had not been what they seemed. In both cases, they had contained an ulterior motive.

This was aggravating. Not many of us like to be caught unaware. For people whose practice is mindfulness, being caught is an old story, however. The catching is the training, and because there seems to be a bottomless reservoir of unmindfulness, enough to last a lifetime, you never run out of training.

To make matters worse (or better, because it's more grist for training), when I stumbled upon my manipulative intent, I also realized a further spiritual implication: I'd taken a vow to try to refrain from false speech. It's one of the Buddhist precepts. Yet, here I was in the thick of it and hadn't realized. For that's what this was, wasn't it, this behavior with an agenda? Does it matter if it's done for what one thinks is someone else's higher good? Does it matter if the words are manipulative but not an outright lie in the way we usually define the term? Is there an essential difference when, in both cases, one's behavior is false? And who's to determine what is another adult's higher good, anyway?

Scriptures and teachers give you guidelines to such issues but not answers. Those you need to find for yourself—and keep on finding them, moment by moment. The late Abbot of Shasta Abbey, the Reverend Master Jiyu Kennett, called Buddhism an "adult religion," because adults are people who take responsibility for their actions, the wise and caring actions as well as the mucky ones.

This one got muckier the more I looked into it. I saw that I had also been lying to myself in a way. For my initial lack of clarity about my motives was self-delusion, and in a broad sense, isn't that a form of lying? There was no blame in this recognition. I didn't castigate myself for blindness; recognizing blindness is simply the stuff of training. Still, I couldn't weasel out of it. When you take seriously the vow to try to refrain from lying, things get subtle.

"Blancheykins" passed away between Mom and me seemingly without an echo. Yet, as I wrote our stories and sang my songs, it whispered, "listen more closely, listen more closely."

Expecting Mother's Day

Mother's Day was not what we expected. Knowing it would be her last, barring a miracle, Mom and I wanted to make it memorable. She didn't want her pain to interfere. With her usual good sense and understatement, she commented, "I'm going to be uncomfortable whether I sit here at home or we go out. Let's go."

We planned a picnic in the park and began discussing the menu the week before. Mom's style was to plan in a leisurely way, whereas I could have decided on the menu in one conversation. How much planning do you need to agree on chicken or cheese sandwiches, carrots and celery and fruit for dessert? And no thought at all was required to include chocolate cookies—they were practically the entree as far as I was concerned. I realized, however, that by giving careful attention to each detail, by embroidering our anticipation, we would prolong our celebration of the occasion. Mother's Day would happen not only on Sunday. We could make it a weeklong event.

There's a gray area here, and I chose to play in it. On a very subtle level, expectations lead to loops of psychological death and rebirth. We usually swing from expectation to expectation—anticipating this or that outcome, and making plans to ensure it. It is human nature to grasp after what one wants and feel let down when events don't meet expectations. Most of us recognize that the new car or dress or house or relationship doesn't remain as intensely gratifying a month (or sometimes even a day or an hour) later. We know that we often become sated and bored with an expectation fulfilled; we're even prepared for the letdown. Many of us, too, are experienced at deferring gratification, postponing enjoyment, for the sake of other people or a greater good. Yet none of this changes the fact that as long as we hold expectations, even subtle ones, we set ourselves up for disappointment and discontent when they aren't fulfilled. This sense of dissatisfaction can be understood as a mind-moment of death. It hurts. Trying to relieve the pain, we sooner or later look to the next expectation. Reaching out and grasping after it becomes a mind-moment of rebirth. Over and over, we grasp, feel pain, and grasp again—unless we learn to drop expectations and to accept what exists.

As one who'd been studying this process for quite some time, I knew that, by creating expectations around our Mother's Day picnic, Mom and I were priming ourselves for disappointment. Nonetheless, I thought making a fuss was a good thing to do. If it poured that day and we had to eat at the kitchen table, I was sure Mom wouldn't be too much more disappointed because we had been anticipating the park for a week. Nor would I. Our picnic planning fell into a gray area between seriously grasping at expectations and refraining. Ours were expectations lightly held, and for me at least, our preparations assumed an aspect of ritual. They were a celebration of the event, beautiful in their own right.

In addition to promoting our mutual expectations, I indulged in a bit of private expecting. I envisioned for our picnic a sylvan scene, the kind you see in Watteau's paintings, minus the finery and the dalliance. The scene came naturally. Mom's chinaware, the set we used when I was a girl—there were still pieces around—was called "Watteau." Its figures, arranged in graceful picnic poses, were fairly fixed in my mind. With every hamburger and string bean, I had ingested Watteau. Trips to art museums over the years augmented the image. Now, it was a composite scene that I envisioned for our picnic—a grassy clearing surrounded by woodlands and, above, billowy clouds bestowing a soft and benevolent glow. But, important point, unlike Watteau's grassy glades, I knew those in Queeny Park had picnic tables.

The unexpected began two days before the occasion. In the mail, Mom received berry plants from an estranged friend. It was a gift that eased a hurt she'd been prepared to die with. She was moved as she gazed at the tender little plants that would outlive her. And the next morning, I found her crying with happiness in her yellow chair, in the kind of emotional response that she seldom permitted herself. Deciding where I should plant the berries became part of our Mother's Day celebration.

Then came the day, hot, sunny, and windy, with fleets of tall clouds at full sail. We found our grassy glade, with picnic tables for our choosing. Eyeing one at the far edge of the clearing in the shade of a shingle oak, we began to make our way over. The wind whacked into us with the force of a lion's roar—

it wasn't the kittensqueak that was skittering about at home. Watteau didn't include that in his landscapes.

Mom, who had grown as frail as a sparrow, slipped her wing into mine for support. Chin tucked in and body bent at a forty-five degree angle, she tottered as we walked toward the table. As though welded into a single being, our combined bulk battled the wind; the bags in my free arm lent extra ballast. Through our linked arms, I felt Mom's unsteadiness as my own, and a visceral sense of being confined to an aged body came over me. It seemed a preview of what it feels like to be truly old.

"That table's far away," I suggested, wanting to end the struggle as soon as possible. "How about this one right here?" I pointed to a nearby table in the sun.

"Fine," Mom said gallantly.

She settled on the bench, while I wrestled the tablecloth, fluttering like a flag, down onto the table and secured the edges with our paraphernalia. Paper plates were hopeless. Instead of setting the table, I sifted through our bags and began to fish out one package at a time.

Three children, a spaniel, and a black Labrador retriever from a nearby party tumbled in the grass as though the sun and wind were made for them. Seemingly carefree, they fit right into my Watteau painting. I glanced at Mom and wondered what she was thinking. "Is she regretting that she's at the end, not at the beginning like them?" I became aware of a vague sense of regret and longing myself, longing not because I wasn't a child any more, but something else, something I couldn't identify, and I didn't try. I handed Mom a sandwich. How did Watteau's gentlefolk *really* feel?

We smiled as we watched the youngsters from behind sunglasses. We smiled and chatted and held our straw hats with one hand to keep the wind, which was making forays under their brims, from snatching them. With the other hand, we ate—first the chicken sandwiches, for which I'd forgotten the lettuce, then the carrots and the celery and the fruit. Knowing paper cups had less chance of remaining upright against the wind than Mom, I poured the sangria after the meal, when we had a hand free to hold the cups. On impulse, I'd picked up a bottle at the supermarket. We'd seen an ad recently, and Mom had said she'd like to try it. Now, as I drank, I found the wine sweeter than I remembered, and I didn't like it. Neither did Mom. The dark chocolate Choco Leibniz cookies were as delicious as I'd anticipated.

Years earlier, during a trip to colonial Williamsburg, Mom had demonstrated her formidable capacity for cheerful endurance. We were both looking forward to dinner one evening at Christiana Campbell's Tavern. Christiana had hosted George Washington, Thomas Jefferson, and other founding fathers, fact enough to make early American history buffs, such as my mother and me, enthusiastic about dining there. Dressing for the occasion, I couldn't find my shoes—not in the closet, under the bed, or in my suitcase. Turning to Mom to enlist her help, I found her laughing, a deep belly laugh so unlike her.

"That's why these shoes hurt so much!" she gasped. "They're yours, not mine!"

In a classic instance of mother-daughter synchronicity, Mom and I, living a thousand miles apart, had bought the same navy pumps—only mine were a couple of sizes smaller than hers. "I wasn't going to say anything. I thought my feet were swollen, and I didn't want to ruin our evening." She was prepared to hobble over to Christiana Campbell's and smile all the way.

Now, our dish-by-dish picnic lunch over, Mom suggested sweetly, "Why don't we go? This bench is getting a little hard."

In addition to the lettuce, I'd forgotten to bring cushions. I was finding the wooden benches uncomfortable myself, but the bigcat wind had burgled my attention and had prevented me from recognizing that, for my frail, smiling mother, sitting on the benches must have been akin to the kind of experience she'd been prepared to endure at Christiana Campbell's Tavern. Now, it occurred to me, too, that the folks in Watteau's paintings probably really wished their pretty party over so they could get up off the hard ground and go home.

As we drove in the shelter of our car up the driveway, past the berry plants by the side of the house and into the garage, Mom said, "This has been a nice Mother's Day."

It wasn't what we had expected, but I think she meant it. And I agreed.

Their Tough Luck

I thought I'd got past my discomfort over Mom's reluctance to talk about dying. I thought I'd settled into accepting that she needed to handle this her way. But accepting wasn't as simple as I thought. For many years, my focus had very explicitly been on solving the great riddle of life and death. Through all the meditation—the aching legs and restlessness and sleepiness and irritation at the person next to me for moving too much—and through all the unsatisfactory little moments of daily life and the satisfactory ones as well, no less than this was the central question.

The answer cannot be found in books or on the lips of teachers. We must find it for ourselves, from the inside. To do that, we need to search beyond the realm of intellectual knowledge, while remaining grounded in the specificity of the present moment. Though there are all sorts of pointers on how to go about this, it's not easy to actually practice it. Each of us needs to do his or her own finding.

What bothered me about Mom, what I just couldn't get past, was that she seemed to have so little interest in the question of life and death. "Why *isn't* she interested?" I wondered time and again. "She doesn't seem to think about her situation much. What's going on?" I suspected that on some level she was in denial, and although I didn't say anything, the possibility pained me.

Around Mother's Day, a slip of the tongue showed me that she thought about dying more than she let on. We were preparing our picnic lunch, and she was standing next to me at the kitchen counter with a loaf of pumpernickel in her hand. Referring to the picnic, she inadvertently said, "When we go to the funeral . . ." Catching herself in mid-sentence, she raised a finger and said, "Oops, sorry, God. Erase that one."

"So she *is* thinking about dying! A lot!" I concluded with an ungenerous sense of satisfaction.

Even deeper than the sense of satisfaction, though, her slip of the tongue stirred in me respect. For it indicated that Mom wasn't denying death. In the face of trying conditions, she was going about her daily affairs, constricted as they were, with cheer and attention. She was looking up, maintaining a bright mind. I marveled at her, and I wondered if I would do as well when my time came.

Mom's ability to be bright in the midst of dismal circumstances was tested the day she moved to the room off of the garage. The move, on a gloomy February day, would have disheartened many people, including me. It was a switch from her room for the past quarter of a century to one she had known as little more than a passageway, the least charming room in the house, the room where she would die. Yet, gazing around her new quarters, Mom commented right away on the snugness of the room, and later she observed enthusiastically, "Now I can look at the pictures!" She was referring to the dozens of family photos she had tacked to a corkboard on the wall.

From her bed, the view of the photos was long distance. Turning to me, she asked for the binoculars. Then, sitting in bed, peering through the lenses, she surveyed her photos, and we talked about the memories they evoked.

Of course, Mom wasn't always cheerful. There were days when her situation overwhelmed her. Then, she would grouse. A clogged drain, the weather, almost anything at all became subject for discontent, as long as it was minor and external. On such days, she invariably apologized, "Don't listen to anything I say today. I'm crabby."

Realizing she was projecting her emotions onto things more acceptable to her than talking about the real issue, I'd assure her, "Don't worry about it, Mom. It's natural to be upset, totally natural." And I wondered again if I wouldn't do a lot worse in her circumstances.

Although I understood her behavior, my soothing reassurances required an act of will because it was hard being around a crabby mother. "Things are tough enough already. Why this too?" I'd grumble to myself. Then I'd commiserate with the caregivers of the world, who have to endure the crabbiness of others, along with all the other problems of life.

One evening I found Mom in bed crying.

"What's wrong, Mom?" The question hardly required an answer since everything was wrong, but tears were so unlike her. I was shaken. I'd seldom seen my mother cry before.

"I hurt. You said it's okay to cry when I need to."

Her explanation contained a half-question, as though, childlike, she needed permission to cry. I gave it to her. "Yes. Yes, cry whenever you want to. It *is* okay," I affirmed softly. Then I asked, "Do you want some methadone?" Needing round-the-clock pain relief now, Mom had graduated to methadone because narcotics in such doses made her retch.

Through her tears and in her misery, she summoned up her energy and replied with force, "Pooh! That won't work!"

Pooh? She was suffering from terminal cancer, and the most she could muster was "pooh"? I, who fairly regularly used stronger language with less provocation, heard cleanness in that "pooh." The problem with foul language is not that it's not nice, but that such language is a form of violence. It is verbal pollution as surely as factory effluents are chemical ones. It affects speaker, listeners, and the environment alike.

In Mom's "pooh," I also heard what was missing. Anger, rage, resentment—those reactions, regarded as classic attitudes toward dying, were ones Mom seemed to have a meager supply of. She hadn't often been angry when she was well. Now that she was dying, anger was still uncharacteristic of her. Toward the end, anger caught up with her, but then, the cause wasn't so much the fact that she was dying, but that she was still alive. She told me a few days before she died, "I've asked God a million times to take me, but still He doesn't do it!"

One day, I told Mom that she was doing a good job at this winding down of her life.

"I am?" she asked with innocent surprise. It hadn't

occurred to her that dying well is as much an art as living well.

"Yes. Many people deny that they're dying or are angry or depressed." I ran through the classic stages of dying, first articulated by Dr. Elisabeth Kübler-Ross.

Mom replied, "It's simple. You see what's inevitable and you accept it."

"Right! But not everybody does that," I commented, casting a quick thought to myself and wondering, yet again, if I would do as well in my time.

With grit and a certain lack of compassion that was understandable in the circumstances, she responded, "That's their tough luck!"

Wild Strawberries
and Good Times

As we drove through the wildlife area with its tangly meadows and woods, close by the Missouri River, Mom exclaimed, "I'm so glad to see this! I'm so glad we came!"

The area was only twenty-five minutes from her house, but she hadn't visited it before. Wildlife wasn't my mother's idea of a good time. And this vista—deciduous Midwest trees and grasses and a scatter of lakes in relatively flat terrain—was unremarkable by most standards. Having seen some of the world's most gorgeous natural places, Mom wasn't easily impressed. When we had driven up California's rugged coast years earlier, she'd conceded, "It's pretty, yes, but it's not like New Zealand."

Right away, I had wanted to set her straight. With effort I'd resisted the urge to reply with a Zen teaching tale. The same story came to mind again during our last months together, but by then, Mom had changed.

The story tells of a man who was chased by a tiger. This man ran as hard as he could, but the tiger kept getting closer and closer. Then he saw a cliff in front of him. It was his only chance. Over the side he scrambled, grabbing a vine as he went. He clutched this vine desperately, because, below the drop was sheer, and above was the ravening animal. As he clung there not knowing what to do, a mouse began to gnaw at the vine. His life collapsed into minutes. Amid this hopelessness, he noticed a cluster of ripe wild strawberries growing nearby. He reached over and picked a berry and ate it. Delicious!

With her time growing short, my mother, like the strawberry eater, seemed to experience her moments more deeply, to appreciate small things in fresh ways, unencumbered by comparisons. She didn't need a Zen story to teach her how. To see wonder in a meadow and woodland scene, she didn't need the marvels of New Zealand. She found wonder in your everyday scribble of branches against the sky.

In healthier times, my mother had been a regular visitor to Missouri Botanical Garden in St. Louis, a world-class garden and horticultural research and education center. She and I had often walked together through its profusion of gardens until our senses grew saturated with beauty. Yet, I never saw her react to any flowers the way she did to a bowl of pedestrian petunias a month before she died.

We had debated which summer flowers I'd plant in the terracotta bowl on the patio table and had settled on petunias. They would do nicely in the sunny location. Before she could see them in bloom, however, she was confined to bed. So, one June day, I carried into her room the rounded bowl filled with deep purple blossoms, each fused petal embellished with a white ray, a bouquet of nodding, starry faces.

"Oh, they're so beautiful!" she gasped, raising her hand to her forehead in an expressive gesture uncharacteristic of her. "So beautiful. Thank you for bringing them in!"

A sponge bath might not be on most people's list of recreational activities, but it became part of Mom's. Lula, a caring, serious woman, attended my mother toward the end. In the mornings, she gave Mom a sponge bath in bed. I knew the bath was prerequisite to the proper start of my mother's day. Fastidious about personal cleanliness, she was restless until she was bathed. I assumed it was simply another item which, once completed, she checked off on her mental daily agenda, for she gave no sign that it was a special pleasure to her.

One morning, however, still in a tranquil mode after meditation, I went to Mom's room to offer hellos and good mornings. Lula was finishing the bath. After quiet greetings all around, Mom looked at us gently and said, "I have such fun when you two are here."

Maybe my ideas about a good time changed a little, too. By the end of June, Mom was comatose much of the time. She had stopped eating and had almost stopped drinking as well. Barbara, our hospice nurse, left on vacation thinking Mom wouldn't be alive when she returned. Yet, a day or two before Barbara was due to return, in a period of alertness, Mom said, "I'd like some wine."

"Why not?" I responded.

My mother was no drinker, but she enjoyed a glass of wine now and then. I'd have happily given her a double shot of whisky if she'd asked.

"I'll just check with hospice to make sure it doesn't conflict with your medicine."

Once we got the go-ahead, I propped Mom up in bed and brought in two glasses of white wine and a plate of potato chips. Putting the plate on her lap and a glass in her hand, I slid in next to her. As we munched and drank side by side, I asked, "How's the wine?"

"The nectar of the gods," she murmured contentedly.

A few nights later when she again awoke briefly, I showed her a prodigious bar of chocolate sent by a friend who knew my predilection for dark chocolate and kindly catered to it. Mom ran her hand down the foot-long length of the hefty bar and said, "I'd like a piece."

A glass of wine, a few chips, a piece of chocolate—have wild strawberries ever tasted better?

Down the Road

One day, in the spring of 1996, when Mom was undergoing chemotherapy, I spent what seemed like all morning waiting for her. I finally heard the garage door open and the car hum to a halt. I rushed out.

"How are you, Mom? You took so long, I was worried!" I fussed over her and hugged her the way a mother would. "I'm fine," she assured me, as though this were just another trip to the supermarket.

It wasn't. It was a very special trip to the supermarket, one on the day after a chemo treatment. Those usually were her bad days, when Mom felt faint and nauseated. But today she had insisted, "I'm okay. I can go alone."

Grocery shopping was an activity my mother relished, and she didn't gladly relinquish the job. Increasingly, however, she'd been forced to, as chemotherapy sapped her energy. Sometimes we went together, and she sat at one of the tables at the front of the supermarket while I shopped. More often, I went by myself.

That day I had acquiesced, reasoning that she was an adult and knew her body's reactions better than I did. So she had

138

driven off happily, and I had stayed home and worried.

Now, as she came into the house, she was quietly pleased by my attentions—I could tell. Then, she dropped into her easy chair and immediately fell into a doze. I went back to the car to bring in the groceries. That small task had never been such a pleasure.

Pleasure or not, my mother was on a one-way street, and it led downhill, and we both knew it. Bit by bit, as the disease worked in her body, the independence and control she so highly prized began to seep away.

Although I was determined that she should keep as much control over her life as possible, what was possible wasn't easy to discern. Her strength fluctuated like mountain weather in the fall—you never knew what was going to be next. I tried to be sensitive to her needs, but, in fact, I was part of the problem. My presence in the house, which she demonstrably appreciated, was a reminder of her waning abilities.

Under any circumstances, more than one woman in a house can cause tension, especially if both are long-term residents. The traditional Chinese character for "peace" is the figure of one woman under a roof; for "cunning," three women under a roof. My mother and I being two, fell between peace and cunning. We tried to respect each other's needs, but we had our moments.

My parents had moved to the house when my sister and I were adults, no longer living with them. The room I now inhabited was a guestroom, set aside mainly for Gail's and my periodic visits. With its two twin beds and not much space for anything else, it was inconveniently arranged for a single steady occupant, especially one who needed to sit there alone sometimes, apart from events elsewhere in the house.

During the first six months that I lived with Mom, when she was taking chemotherapy, the inconvenience of the bedroom pestered me, but it seemed fairly unimportant. Later, when I returned for the duration, the desire to make changes became insistent. Each time I put books and papers on the extra bed for want of other storage space, each time I sat on the floor in meditation squeezed between the two beds, the desire for change mounted. It mounted, and then it collided with the certainty that Mom would find changes disruptive. They would be a challenge in her ordered domain.

I meditated with the dilemma, using a Buddhist technique. I formulated the question when I began to meditate. Should I rearrange the room? Then, without trying to figure out an answer, I let the question hover. If I could get enough space from the bedlam often happening in my mind, I knew the answer would be clear. This took time because bedlam is engrossing.

Gradually, however, it did get clear. I was there to support my mother. Any changes I made to the décor would have the opposite effect, and, in any case, they weren't essential to my well being. You can't live in a monastery for any length of time without loosening your attachment to décor, at least a little.

Nonetheless, my presence needed to be honored, too. I wasn't Cinderella in her pre-prince days, sitting by the hearth tending the fire but otherwise a supernumerary in the household. Wholesale changes to the décor throughout the house weren't in question, but changes to the room I lived in seemed legitimate. And they wouldn't affect accommodations for Gail,

Bruce, or other guests, who could stay in the master bedroom now that Mom was using the room off of the garage.

The first change was trivial—on purpose. A small change was less likely to offend Mom. I removed from the dresser a tall, decorative, brass-plated candlestick with a glass protector patterned after an early American design. In its place, I created an arrangement of graceful sycamore branch ends, lotus pods, and dried, flowering boysenberries—an arching composition in browns, which I placed in a clear glass carafe.

"Simple and beautiful," I thought, pleased with the effect against the sky-blue walls. I also removed a bunch of small, nineteenth-century prints whose presence on the walls felt like an intrusion.

Mom was less than pleased. Coming into the room at my invitation to view the flower-and-twig creation, she composed a little smile and looked away. Then, remembering her good manners, she uttered a taut "that's nice."

Her response, like a bucket dropped into a well, splashed deep inside and disturbed me. And it didn't stop disturbing me for the rest of the day and the next. The echo called to me and insisted that something here needed looking into. Interesting how uneasiness is a teacher if we heed it.

I looked. I saw that I hadn't talked with Mom about making changes because I wanted to avoid unpleasantness. Because I felt embattled, I'd acted unilaterally, and my actions contained an element of, well, cowardice. And hostility.

Making the changes wasn't a problem—I felt on firm ground there—but the way I'd made them was. I needed to be more sensitive to Mom's feelings. To explain why I wanted to change some things, to do it without rancor, and to bring her into the process, that's what was needed.

I waited until after dinner the next evening when we both were relaxed, presumably. As Mom sat with her mug of regular coffee and I with mine of decaf, pinching the handle between my thumb and forefinger, I began. In what I hoped was a casual tone, I said, "You know, Mom, now that I'm living in the back room, I'm finding a few problems there."

It got easier as I went. As I let go of my defensiveness, Mom let go of hers and listened. Then we began to consult, not all at once, but over the next few weeks. We talked about removing the extra bed and donating the mattress and frame to charity, adding a bookcase to store items accumulating on the bed, and moving in a cricket chair from another room to give me a place apart to sit and read.

By the time I brought home cushions for the cricket chair—I brought two or three for discussion—Mom was enthusiastic. We chose flounced, blue-flowered chintz ones that fit prettily in the room. I returned the others, and we were both pleased. Many times thereafter, Mom assured me, "This is your house, too." Although it didn't feel like mine, I was glad to hear her say so.

One duty Mom happily yielded was cooking. "You be chief chef and I'll be sous-chef," she offered. I like to cook, but I wondered if chief chef mightn't become a doubtful honor.

In fact, it was fine. While Mom was well enough, we each usually made our own breakfasts and lunches. Dinner, then, was the occasion to exercise my responsibilities. The dinner menu was a daily topic. She often raised it after breakfast: "What'll we have for dinner?"

"Mom," I complained, "we just had breakfast. How can we think about dinner?"

My frequent preference was to figure out dinner as I browsed the refrigerator for possibilities at 5:45. We learned to compromise, though, discussing the menu early enough to satisfy her need for closure and late enough for me to begin to feel the topic warranted attention. And we enjoyed it. In fact, I purposely tried to make it fun. Sometimes I teased her, asking after breakfast, "What do you think about dinner?"

She'd laugh and say, "Now look who's talking about dinner early!"

Discussing the menu and proposing new dishes helped entice her to eat at a time when she was losing her appetite. "Here's something interesting—a broccoli-Swiss frittata," I commented one afternoon, a vegetarian cookbook at my elbow.

"What's a frittata?" she asked predictably. This gave us a chance to discuss Italian-style omelets, a subject with which I'd become conversant only five minutes earlier. We both wanted to try one.

The challenges and fun in learning to share did not, however, change the prospect, waiting down the road, that Mom's condition would decisively worsen. The time would come, not too long from now, when she would have to relinquish everything except the space she occupied in her bed. Then she'd have to relinquish that, too.

Mom strove to maintain her routines as long as possible— reading in her recliner much of the day, watching news in the evening, listening to an hour of classical music in bed before she took her sleeping pills. Toward the end, only her will dragged her disfigured body from bed in the morning. And her will dragged her to the commode by her bedside at night.

Until the night she fell. I'm not usually awake at 2:30 a.m., and from my room at the opposite end of the house, I usually couldn't hear what was happening in hers. But that June night I was awake, and I did hear. I wonder at that now. Hearing commotion in her room, I went in and helped her off the floor.

"I guess we're down the road," Mom said as I lifted her.

Because her decline had been gradual and fluctuating, we were reluctant to admit that "down the road" had arrived. Now, there was no denying it.

Still, Mom was determined to hang on to a last particle of independence, insisting she could manage alone at night. But soon her weakening body began to give way day and night, and she was confined to bed.

Down the road—that's where I was too. There was no choice; I had to face it. I needed full-time help. I'd known it would come to this, but accepting wasn't easy.

Mom didn't want strangers in her house. From the beginning, she welcomed help from Jennifer, a hospice aide who came three times a week to bathe her. She explained that she didn't want to burden me. "You're busy enough already."

I think modesty was a factor, too. She preferred that a stranger see her nakedness rather than I, though as time went on, she had to abandon that reservation. Mom looked forward to Jennifer's visits. Chatting with this kind young woman offered diversion in her limited daily routine. However, the prospect of full-time nursing care, someone who would be in the house all of the time, someone—actually several people—whose ways she'd have to adjust to, was altogether without appeal.

I was ambivalent myself. Mom's objections weighed on me. Although she thoughtfully assured me that she understood I couldn't manage alone anymore, I was assailed by an inner sense that I should be able to. Guilt. Mom's preference, cost— home nursing care would be expensive—but most of all, my own ego made me hesitate. I cherished a half-hidden image of myself as competent, not simply your average, everyday competence, but competence writ large, where it got interesting. I saw myself as a lone ranger out at the frontier battling adversity, and, from that perspective, the prospect of hiring round-the-clock nursing assistance was repugnant. It was thoroughly inconsistent with my self-image.

A baby monitor wasn't, however. I tried it—sleeping with a baby monitor in my room with the other half of the hook-up in Mom's so that I could hear if she called me at night. I found that the static and the sound of her movements and her breathing prevented me from sleeping well. They showed me that young parents perform heroic deeds each night and that a baby monitor wasn't for me.

So I hired full-time help, still feeling guilty. It was as though I'd never heard of the basic rule of caregiving, the rule that says caregivers must take care of themselves. Soon afterward, I asked Lula, who had been at this work for more than thirty years, "Do families usually get full-time care for a dying patient at this stage?" Her "yes" was a big relief, as if she had given me permission to let go of my guilt.

Wrong to begin with, and wrong at the end, and the funny thing is, I knew it all along. I was caught in delusional thinking. My resistance to asking for help sprang from an unreal expectation about myself, which is a form of egotism. And it was reinforced by false references to what other people might think. No one was blaming me for asking. Moreover, by reacting to the imagined opinions of others, I was not grounding my behavior in the needs of the situation, which is the true grounding place.

I told myself, "My guilt is my choice. I created it, and I can let it go."

But this piece of wisdom had no effect against my delusion, which had all the strength of an old oak beam. Lula's words allowed me to let go of the discomfort of guilt, but I didn't let go of my super-self image. It persists in one form or another today. Maybe I'll be able to drop it someday, someday down the road.

Bad Car Karma

It started in chapel at the beginning of June, a month and a half before Mom died. As I was meditating there, on the grounds of a Catholic monastery, I heard a man behind me ask quietly, addressing all within, "Who has a black Nissan Sentra?"

I knew immediately what that was about. "Oh, well, I was almost through meditating anyway," I thought ruefully, arising to inspect the damage.

Bad car karma had reached right into this hallowed setting where I'd gone to seek a refuge. I use the word "karma" loosely. "Karma," the law of cause and effect, strictly applies only to the results of our intentional acts. This accident had nothing to do with my intentions. I wasn't even present for it. But the term is often used loosely, as it is here, to refer to any event or events that occur in one's life.

At the auto shop a few days later while waiting for an assessment of the repair costs, which Mr. Maxwell was offering to pay, he and I made amiable introductions. I learned about his first gun, squirrel hunting, and his lumber business. He learned why I was in St. Louis.

Over the talk-show banter that swarmed out of the television and buzzed around us in the waiting room, he said with kind concern, "I'll pray for your mother." When I told Mom about his prayers, she smiled—no matter he was a Catholic and she a Jew. "I need them," she said.

Then, there was the second accident. It happened in the high hills outside of the little, old-timey town of Las Vegas, New Mexico. Early in June when Mom was still ambulatory, I happily took a week's vacation, time for myself the caregiver, in honor of hardships past and in recognition of what was yet to come. Gail came to town and stayed with Mom while I visited my friend Kee.

In a car I'd rented, Kee and I drove up to the United World College. The mission of this two-year institution, which is to foster global cooperation, seemed at odds with its remote location, snuggled into tall, forested ridges, keeping its distance from the world. Up there, backing the car to turn around on what resembled a path more than a road, I heard "clonk", and we were stuck. I didn't want to know why. Instead, holding my breath, I pressed the gas pedal hard. It worked—the car lurched free. Then, I got out to look, and I found that the left rear tire was slashed, ripped by a metal post that protruded bayonet-like at a forty-five degree angle from the underbrush. Just behind that was an overgrown culvert.

Grounds personnel, implementing the college's global mission locally, kindly changed the tire for the spare. But back in town at a service station, where I purchased a new tire, the attendant informed us that the sway bar near the tire had been bent. That, too, would eventually have to be replaced.

I turned to Kee and said, "We need to look at the half-full side of this glass. A little farther back and the rear half of the car would have been in the culvert. So we're lucky."

I didn't feel lucky, though. It could have happened to anyone, this accident, but it hadn't. It had happened to me. And it had happened less than a week after the accident with Mr. Maxwell.

"That's two," I thought, sensing a pattern.

I knew better. I knew the accidents were unconnected and that I needed to take them one by one. I was creating something extra here, a notion that I was being victimized by a punitive universe. Spiritual training is a long effort of learning to see clearly, without imposing our fears, superstitions, or wishful thinking. "Life as it is, the only teacher" as Zen teacher Charlotte Joko Beck points out. This second accident had happened because I hadn't been mindful. I'd been dividing my attention between driving and talking with Kee, and all the while oppressed by deep-body tensions that had accumulated over the months of caregiving. Signs along that sketchy road warning drivers not to enter hadn't contributed to my peace of mind, either. With every sign I passed, I felt heavier, and the need to turn back grew more insistent. It was as though I were driving with the emergency break on. Then, clonk, we were stopped in our tracks. The internal drag I was feeling seemed to have materialized in the form of a metal post. Maybe it wasn't a hostile universe, at all. Could my mind have created that post?

The problem of car insurance added additional weight to the event. When I'd gone to live at the monastery a couple of years earlier, I'd sold my car and cancelled my insurance. In

St. Louis, as I became sole driver of my mother's car, we placed the car in joint ownership, but we left the insurance policy in her name, with a provision covering me. I was uncomfortable with the arrangement, knowing that any accident I had would be registered against her policy. Changing the policy was probably as simple as a phone call, but I never got around to it.

Now, the mangled tire sharpened my concern. I didn't want this accident to be reported on Mom's record, though I knew she'd never drive again. Nor did I want it to affect the application for my own insurance, which seemed more urgent than ever.

"Who's your insurance company?" the agent at Alamo Rental in Albuquerque asked when I returned the car and told him about the accident. His assurances that they wouldn't need to contact the company if I paid for damages didn't prevent me from storing the worry in my mind. It was a "what if," something that wouldn't likely happen, but the possibility could niggle at me if I let it.

Car insurance had to wait. Immediately after I returned to St. Louis, Mom grew worse. That's when number three occurred. During an emergency trip to the pharmacy one night to pick up disposable diapers, I made a wide right turn—for sure my attention wasn't on driving—and I hit an oncoming car. That jolted me into the present.

Standing in a parking lot under the dim neon lights of a closed-up store, the young driver and I inspected our cars. He and his vehicle seemed totally unscathed, not a scratch. Mine had what would amount to over $1,500 worth of damage. I was numb. I felt oppressed not only by the damage to the car, but also by a sense that bad car karma was after me. I, who seldom had car accidents, now had three in a row, each more serious than the last. "What did I do to deserve this?" I moaned to myself.

I didn't really believe God was peering down from heaven and targeting me to see how much I could handle at this most trying time. I understood that there is a universal nature, That Which Is, but not a personal god who watched my deeds, keeping score, to punish or reward me. I knew these auto accidents were merely the operation of impersonal forces. It was just the way things had happened. And yet . . . yet something more than ordinary seemed to be going on. Things were working in some mighty funny ways, as far as I was concerned.

"Business or pleasure?" the insurance agent asked the next day, taking preliminary information about the accident over the phone.

"Neither," I responded. "My mother is dying, and I was on my way to the pharmacy to pick up supplies for her. There wasn't an ounce of pleasure in it."

In my mind, I saw her click the "pleasure" option on her computer screen. Deciding I may as well get the bad news, I asked about the effect this accident would have on my forthcoming insurance application.

"Probably none. Now, if you had a second accident in the next six months, then you'd have a problem."

Quickly I sent a stern affirmation to Alamo Rental in Albuquerque: "You will keep your promise!" I commanded. It was a tactic to make any Buddhist master shudder. Spiritual training cultivates the power of realistic thinking, but not manipulative thinking that seeks to rearrange life in order to suit oneself.

"Okay, this little affirmation takes care of past transgressions," I continued, only half-joking to myself. Then, still beset by a sense of victimization by hostile cosmic forces, I turned to the future and wondered if a fourth accident, possibly a catastrophic one this time, were waiting to happen soon.

I told Mom about the first accident, which seemed innocuous, but I didn't mention numbers two and three. There was no point to it. Nor did I tell her about the car I'd rented after the third event while ours was in the shop for repairs. However, because around this time she'd sensed, without actually seeing it, that a tree had fallen in the yard, I kept wondering if she'd intuit the car accidents too. I kept expecting her to ask me why someone else's car was in the garage just outside the door to her room. But she never did.

Catastrophizing

When I telephoned the Abbey during the last spring of Mom's life, the monk taking the call asked if I had an emergency. It was a standard question for incoming calls from congregation members requesting spiritual guidance.

I paused as I ran through my issues to see if any fit into the "emergency" category. Then I responded, "Well, if my mother dies tonight, I guess that would be an emergency, but otherwise, no—I'm just going along."

As I spoke, I noted with surprise that before I had begun caring for my mother, I would have considered almost everything I was experiencing as a caregiver to be an emergency. Now I wasn't sure what an emergency was.

But soon thereafter, I was faced with a situation that seemed to have the makings of a real emergency, and I immediately expanded it into one. It began quietly one evening in late June. As I sat reading in Mom's room at the end of a long day, I heard, *plop, plop, plop.* I looked behind me to find the source of the squishy sound. Once, twice, I glanced at the large bouquet of lemon lilies on the desk, sent by my friend Jane.

"Maybe the petals are falling, and they're heavier than they look," I speculated. Not a petal stirred.

I read a little longer, while Mom lay unresponsive, as she had been most of that day. Then I left the room, forgetting about the mystery sound.

When I came back in, what had become a steady dribble from the ceiling hit me on the head.

The tubing in the air-conditioning pump, located in the attic above the room, had clogged the preceding summer, and we'd had to poke a hole in the ceiling to let the water drain. The stream had lasted hours, so this rivulet shouldn't have been a surprise. We had known that the antiquated system was likely to fail at any time, but Mom was too sick to consider replacing it. In recent months, her ability to cope with maintenance matters around the house had declined markedly. She had lost elasticity, and even minor household problems had become more than she could countenance.

I scurried around, moving a bookcase out from under the flow and placing buckets to catch it. Greater than my concern to protect the furniture and floor, however, was a driving need to prevent Mom from finding out what was happening. I called into service a handful of rags. Stuffed into the buckets to muffle the sound of the falling water, they became my co-conspirators. We would do our best to keep Mom from worrying.

Her hearing was deteriorating, so there was a real chance the rags would work, that she wouldn't hear the water when she became alert again. I hoped too, against reason, that she wouldn't notice the buckets on the floor. But her eyesight was unimpaired, and the buckets were only five feet from her bed.

"Well, at least it's not dripping right on her," I sighed, trying for a moment to see the bright side of the situation.

Then, my mind broke bounds and took off, lunging after a vision of disaster: a fried air-conditioning system in the ninety-plus-degree heat with humidity to match meant I'd have to call an ambulance. Mom would have to be moved to a hospital while the system was being replaced. And who knows how much that would cost.

As I catastrophized, the disaster grew worse and worse. The disruption could kill her—a disturbed death in a sterile hospital, wrenched unwillingly and unexpectedly at her weakest moment from the home she loves. All my efforts to allow her to die in peaceful circumstances seemed about to crash against a little spent motor and some rusty tubes. I stood there, buckets at my feet, expanding on the grim scenario and becoming increasingly agitated. My mother was comatose and motionless, and I was anything but.

Making a realistic appraisal of a situation and its possible consequences is only common sense. But there's a fine line, so readily crossed, between appraising and wallowing in things that might never happen, in upsetting oneself unnecessarily and abandoning the effort to be mindful of things as they truly are in the present moment.

Pulling myself from the catastrophe I was devising, I called the air-conditioning service. Kevin, who was on emergency duty that night, arrived at the house in less than an hour.

He needed to see the leaky ceiling, so I led him into

Mom's room. He tromped through as quietly as his work boots permitted, observed the leak, glanced at Mom unconscious, then tromped out the other door and into the garage, where the hatch to the attic was located. Under normal circumstances, the activity would have awakened her. The garage door squealed open on its rollers, not forty feet from Mom's bed. Each shrieking inch of the door's progress made me contract, as though my insides could absorb the noise and keep her from hearing. Kevin brought a ladder in and clambered up. While he observed from on high, he called down to me to turn the system off, then on, then off again.

Back and forth through Mom's room, between the garage and the control dial in the dining room, I tiptoed, desperately wanting her not to hear. Tiptoeing was ludicrous in view of the ruckus we were making on the other side of the door, but all I could think of was that I didn't want to disturb her. I knew that even when people are unconscious and oblivious of their environment, they frequently hear what is happening around them, and they remember afterwards. That's why, each time I returned to the garage to stand at the base of the ladder and shout up to Kevin, "Okay, it's off," then, "It's on," then "It's off again," I tried to shout very quietly.

When Kevin came down, we moved out to the driveway, away from the house, to confer.

"The tubing was clogged, but I blew it out. It'll work now," he reported. "But the dripping from the ceiling could last a couple of days."

Uh-oh. I'd been counting on removing the buckets before Mom regained consciousness.

He continued, "And even after it stops, it could happen again at any time." He explained that the drip tray under the pump was leaking, but it was pointless to replace it without replacing the dilapidated pump as well. The cost of a real fix?

"Seventeen to twenty-three."

"Seventeen to twenty-three thousand dollars!" I nearly shouted, incredulous.

Prepared to hear the worst, that is what I heard. With my attitude shaping my perception and braced for probable calamity, my thoughts leapt to the astronomical figures rather than the common sense ones.

"No, seventeen hundred dollars to twenty-three hundred dollars," Kevin quietly responded.

Deciding there was nothing to do except hope the air-conditioning system outlived my mother, I thanked him, paid him, and said good-bye. And I carried my calamitous mind-set back into Mom's room.

Walking in, I warily eyed the buckets on the floor, and a new worry shot through me. What if Dovie, the nursing aide who was just coming on night duty, walked into the room in the middle of the night, tripped on one of the buckets, fell, and broke a leg or an arm? I could imagine myself doing that if I had to rush into the room in an emergency. When Dovie arrived, the first thing I said to her, my mind racing, was, "Are you bonded?" "No, but don't worry," she quietly assured me, patting my arm. "I won't sue."

By the next morning, Mom was alert. She asked innocently, "Is something wrong with the air conditioner?"

The leak from the ceiling mercifully had stopped, and

I'd removed the buckets, though I hadn't yet returned the bookcase to its former position.

"No, Mom. Everything's fine," I assured her calmly, as though my imagination had not run amok, as though I had not stowed my spiritual training and plunged into the havoc of a manufactured emergency.

Not a Word

"Why am I in bed?"

It wasn't a question seeking an answer. Mom flung at me an accusation: she was being wrongly used.

"What am I doing here day after day?" she demanded one morning in July, a week or two before she died.

Her tone took me aback. Was this belligerence coming from my mother? In the past few weeks, she'd been increasingly angry, but so deep-rooted was my expectation that she'd display her usual even disposition that each departure surprised me. In the circumstances, anger was more than understandable, but I'd come to rely on her good nature. Now that it was absent, I almost felt she was letting me down.

I didn't know what to say. Sweet evasion? Silence, pretending I didn't hear? Or the self-centered view? "Mom, you're not *supposed* to be like this"? It was one of those situations where nothing I said was going to be right.

Honesty seemed the best recourse. "You're dying, Mom. Don't you know?" I said as gently as I could. She'd been in bed four weeks all told, and for the past three, she'd barely eaten or drunk. It was a wonder she was still alive.

"No, I *don't* know," she asserted. "I feel foolish. If the doctor came and saw me in bed, he'd laugh."

Our lines were drawn. I couldn't turn back.

"No, he wouldn't laugh. He knows you're dying. Barbara and I know it. And it's important that you should, too."

"Well, I don't!" She held her ground.

"You've been lucky, Mom, because your mind has been clear. And you haven't been in a lot of pain for the most part. The medicine is taking care of that."

Then—this one took courage—I continued, "But your body is dying. God is putting His hand on your body and letting you know your time is near. You need to listen to your body."

Something was loosening a flow of words on a subject we had seldom discussed at length. "You've got a strong mind, Mom. It's used to making decisions about what to do and where to go and what to keep and what to give away. They were good decisions, and you followed them, but now things are changing. Now your body isn't obeying your mind anymore."

"What makes you so smart?" she snapped.

Good question! "How could I be saying these things? How did I get into this?" I asked myself. I agonized over this confrontation that was sending chunks of tension hurtling through my body like a train at night. I didn't want to be here. I searched for a deep-down reply, knowing my response needed to be as bald as her question. I had to say the truth.

"I know. . . ." I stopped, groping to express it in a way she'd relate to and, not finding one, deciding to be blunt. "I know because I've meditated for years. From my meditation I've learned to understand things in ways that I wouldn't otherwise."

I was commenting not on my observation that she was dying—that took no special skill to discern. I was referring to my ability to meet her question honestly and to respond from the deepest place I knew. It wasn't easy. Despite my long yearning to talk with Mom about dying, I wasn't practiced at it. Although I had frequently urged her to share her feelings and thoughts, I had expected no response, and I had seldom got one. I understood, however, that it was important to let her know that she could talk with me if she wanted to.

Then, lo, one morning she had raised the subject on her own. It was March, four months before she died, and we were sitting in the living room looking at photos I'd taken the week before when my cousin Vicki had visited. As we sat on the couch, the pictures spread between us, Mom gazed around the room, at the windows hung with old-fashioned ruffly curtains, at the spinet that hadn't been played since Gail and I were girls, the parquet floor embellished with an oval, Wedgwood blue area rug edged with a white floral pattern and a coffee stain that no amount of cleaning could remove. She was silent a moment, then looking at me, she quietly said, "I love this room. It's just the way I want it to be. I'm going to have to leave this soon." Because there seemed to be nothing to say, I simply reached for her hand and squeezed it.

Now, as I sat by her bedside, a rivulet of words poured forth. In response to her challenge, I continued, "No one can make you truly know what's happening except you. You do know already, but your mind is in the way. You need to let yourself know what you know. It's a gift only Blanche can give to Blanche."

After a moment's silence, Mom replied, "How do I get my mind out of the way?"

"She's more receptive than I thought. Here's my chance to share with her!" I exclaimed inwardly. Then, I checked myself, "Not too much detail, lightly, lightly—let her absorb and react as she will."

I spoke lightly and simply—quite eloquently, I thought—explaining how, by meditating, she could reach for a place of deeper peace. And then, as I spoke, thrilling to the clarity of the words, my mother fell asleep.

Looking back on our conversation, I realize that Mom was delirious. The possibility hadn't occur to me at the time because she had sounded coherent. No raving or mumbling or tossing about—behaviors I associated with delirium. I realize now though, that if I'd repeated her comments to her later, she wouldn't have remembered a word she'd said. Nor one I had.

Neither Miracles nor Magic

My sense is—I'll never know for sure—that my words and the energy healing I did pulled Mom back from where she was slipping away to. They reeled her in like a fish on a silver line, drew her back from some zone beyond the precincts of common knowing. Ultimately, the choice to return was hers, of course. But I'm not sure I did her a service.

In April, Barbara told us that a hospice social worker would be visiting soon.

"Uh-oh," I thought, remembering an occasion early on when another hospice social worker had paid us a call. She'd stayed only a short time, talking first with me, then trying to talk with Mom. But Mom was retching and had waved her out of the room. The social worker said she would return, but she never did. Mom and I later joked that we had been a flop.

The problem stemmed, I'm sure, less from Mom's helpless lack of cordiality than from my attitude. I welcomed a social worker's assistance for Mom if she wanted it, but *I* didn't want to be part of someone's caseload. My spiritual training, periodic phone conversations with Reverend Master Eko at Shasta Abbey, and the support of friends, family, and hospice, personified by Barbara, would see me through, or nothing would. Sometimes, I thought nothing would. A social worker, no matter how skilled and well-intentioned, would be an unnecessary addition to my life, a burden, in fact.

So when Barbara spoke about a new social worker, wariness prickled. I felt my belly go tight. Then, she mentioned that Kate did Healing Touch, a form of energy healing.

"Well, that's a different story!" I thought. "That's interesting. Very interesting."

I'd heard about energy healing now and then, but I didn't know much about it. I felt a strong connection, though. I'd often put my hands on people and wounded animals in an intuitive gesture of healing.

Once in New Mexico, I picked up a junco that was lying dazed on the ground after it had hit the window of a trailer in the desert where I was staying. Cupping the little frail body in my hands, its beak quivering with shock, I meditated for I don't know how long, maybe ten or fifteen minutes. I felt a stirring and gently opened my hands. The creature remained still a moment, its beak now relaxed; then it hopped out to a stubble a few feet away. It perched there, gathering strength. Then it flew, flew back onto my hands that had cradled it—just an instant, just a touch—and off it soared. I was stunned. This was the bird's expression of gratitude!

It took me a moment to realize what had happened. But I never forgot it, this communication between me and this precious wild thing. In a meditative state where my effort had been to allow the walls of my ego, my separateness, to dissolve, I had offered up a pure intention on behalf of this small being. It was the essence of energy healing, though I didn't know it then. And the bird had responded.

Are we so different from all that is out there? Is there an "out there?"

I watched covertly for Mom's reactions while Barbara explained that Healing Touch is a natural form of healing that usually is done just outside the body, in a person's energy field.

"'Energy field'—that's a weird one," I thought, trying to assess Mom's inner response, knowing the term would jar her. My mother was impassive.

Barbara continued, "By balancing a person's energy, Healing Touch can relieve physical pain and tension. A lot of times it works on nonphysical levels, too."

A knot squeezed my belly, and I hunched forward slightly as I waited for Mom's decision. I wished, very much wished, her to have the treatment. In fact, as Barbara spoke I knew that I wanted to learn to do it and that I had always wanted to.

"It has to be Mom's choice. She has to want it, no urging from me," I cautioned myself.

"Okay. Why not?" Mom said.

My body relaxed. I felt sure Mom agreed because the suggestion had come from Barbara, a medical professional whom she respected, a trusted guide through this world of endings. Maybe, too, her disease had made her more receptive. Earlier,

Mom likely would have rejected the unorthodox treatment out of hand.

Before Kate arrived, I investigated local organizations that offered Healing Touch training. I found that the only course in town, which was offered through the nursing college at Washington University's medical school, wouldn't be run until the fall. I planned to enroll, but I knew fall would be too late to help Mom. She wouldn't be alive by fall.

In the meantime, I signed up for a soon-to-be-held course in introductory Reiki, which was offered through a private center that taught healing arts. Reiki, with origins in the Far East, is a form of energy healing older than Healing Touch. Though they have somewhat different modalities, Reiki and Healing Touch, which was developed by American nurses in recent decades, are based on a common principle. They both hold that, by helping balance a person's energy, healing work can promote emotional and spiritual healing, and sometimes it can facilitate a physical cure.

For many people, the concept of energy healing smacks of the bizarre, if not outright sorcery. Others find blasphemous any effort to practice the laying on of hands, for that was a means through which Jesus Christ worked miracles. Scientific research, however, is finding that there is nothing miraculous about the human energy field. We each have one, and it can be measured. Studies are beginning to provide quantitative data showing that human energy can be modulated by ordinary people trained in energy healing. Some of us need no convincing.

A few days before Kate was to arrive, Mom fell and fractured a bone in her wrist. Invaded by cancer, her bones were weakening, and we knew to expect a growing number of breaks. Her right wrist and hand were wrapped in a soft splint; her swollen fingers resembled little sausages.

"It doesn't hurt," Mom maintained brightly.

She had a high tolerance for pain, so I don't know if she was telling the truth, or if she was being stoic. What clearly did hurt though was her jaw. Even Mom couldn't mask that pain.

"On a scale of one to ten, how much does your jaw hurt?" I asked. Barbara had taught me how to assess pain, though she cautioned that one person's ten might be another's eight or six or four.

"It's a ten," Mom replied.

I believed her. The radiating pain in her jaw was a sign that the cancer was spreading from its primary site in the bones to her central nervous system. It had been sending her to bed for weeks. Dilaudid, the medication we were reserving for strong pain, barely touched it. As we waited for Kate that day, I knew that Healing Touch was facing a tough case. Maybe too tough.

"Please let this work. Let this help Mom somehow." I sent out a prayer to the universe.

Kate came and worked, and I watched with such obvious interest that she explained what she was about. Within an hour of her departure, however, pains began to blaze up Mom's arm, from the fractured wrist to her shoulder. That hadn't happened before. She took Dilaudid and went to bed.

"Oh, no, that's it!" I groaned inwardly. I was concerned about Mom's pain, but, truly, at the moment I was more distressed by the failed healing effort. A door that had begun to open slammed shut before there was a chance to step inside.

An hour later, Mom was up again. "I feel much better!" she declared.

Remarkably, the pain in her arm had disappeared. Examining her fingers, we noticed the swelling had subsided. They were normal-sized now. Most stunning of all, the searing pain in her jaw was completely gone. And it never returned with the old severity. We both were sure this wasn't the effect of the Dilaudid.

It was a lesson in the way energy works. Sometimes the shift in energy caused by healing techniques can result temporarily in new pain, as old, unbalanced energy patterns gradually transform.

Mom became a believer. Neither of us expected a physical cure for her cancer—no magic—but we realized that energy healing could mean something else besides a physical cure. It could ease her final months.

Kate began to visit once a week, sometimes more often. She generously invited me to participate in the healing sessions, instructing me as we went along. Mom didn't mind being a guinea pig. To the contrary, she liked the idea that these lessons would enable me to work with her between Kate's visits.

"What did you feel?" Kate asked after I had passed my hands through Mom's energy field from head to toes. "Was any place warmer than others?"

"Well, I'm not sure, but it seems to me her legs are warmer here." I pointed diffidently.

"Trust your sense of it," she counseled. Repeatedly, Kate

encouraged me to trust what I was experiencing and not to worry if I felt nothing.

"Energy is subtle, and you'll get more sensitive to it as you go. Just trust. You won't do harm."

She couldn't have given me better advice. As a beginner, I needed encouragement. Yet, there was a deeper understanding to be gained here. A healing practitioner needs training, of course, and in a formal sense, I was just starting. The essence of energy healing, however, lies in the fact that the healer exerts no personal power, for the healer is not an actor but an agent for a higher healing energy. Feelings of inadequacy as well as those of adequacy are hindrances that get in the way of the work to be done. The healer must work from a place of clarity, a place unclouded by self-images, whether positive or negative.

I knew this from my Buddhist practice, but I've had to keep learning it over and over, so prone is the ego to slide back and forth between confidence and lack of it. To act from the clear middle—which is not a linear in-betweenness, but a dimension outside the scale—is to not act at all. Rather, it is to allow oneself to become an agent.

And that was just the beginning. I found that training in energy healing was a discovery in a new context of many truths I'd already learned. I was amazed. I completed my first course in Reiki with wide eyes and quiet excitement. "Here, too! Here, too!" The unfolding of the course was like a beam of light illuminating a landscape I was already familiar with! Revealed was the heart of Buddhism applied to energy healing.

I told Tom, the Reiki master whose sensitive manner of

teaching conveyed deep spirituality, "I'll be back for more."

For Mom, the Reiki and Healing Touch I did almost daily for the next two and a half months meant, first of all, a time for us to share. She expanded under the attention and the touch of my hands. I'd often put my arms around her and kissed her, but this was a different kind of relating. It was a connection that carried us out beyond the emotional fields of our mother-daughter roles into a region where two beings met in relative stillness and where I, the practitioner, offered a heart's-wish for her highest good, whatever that good might be.

The razzle-dazzle results of the first Healing Touch session with Kate weren't matched again. That was too much to expect, I guess. But sometimes Mom was surprised by what happened when I worked. "I feel waves rising from my legs!" she exclaimed one day while I was using a Healing Touch technique called Unruffling. "Right there, below my knees," pointing to her shins, which were misshapen by tumors.

"I've never felt anything like it before. Keep doing what you're doing."

I left Mom's room where I'd been reading and walked back to mine. I needed a break. Barbara was due to arrive soon, and I wanted some time to be alone first.

It was late in Mom's illness. She was bedridden and unconscious most of the time. Earlier in the day, Lula and I had noticed that Mom was unusually quiet. She'd been experiencing apnea, periods without breathing, and I knew that at any time she might not breathe again. But I didn't think it would happen that day.

I wasn't in my room long before Lula came to the door, held out a hand, and quietly said, "Come on."

I was irritated. "Barbara can get started without me," I thought, assuming that Barbara had arrived and I hadn't heard her.

"I'll be there in a few minutes, Lula. I'm not ready now," I snapped.

She turned without comment and walked back down the hall.

Suddenly I knew: Mom wasn't breathing. I raced to Mom's room, overtaking Lula on the way.

I looked and looked at Mom and searched for movement, any movement however slight, peering at her as though by intensity I could conjure it into being. "She's been like this for the past five minutes," Lula whispered.

She put her arms around me and we embraced.

As we stood wrapped in this hug, a knowing welled up and spilled all though me like water over the top of a dam: "Don't stand here. Help Mom."

"There's something I need to do for her," I told Lula, and I pulled away.

Facing Mom, I was aware that my hands, my whole body, were trembling. I tried to calm myself.

"Mind of meditation, put yourself in the mind of meditation," I sternly instructed myself. I tried to, but I didn't do a very good job. My body wasn't listening.

I started, shaking. Bending over Mom, I whispered in her ear, "I love you, Mom. Have a safe journey."

I sensed rather than saw a stirring. Almost imperceptibly, something seemed to shift in her body. Then I began Reiki and Healing Touch, wondering as I worked how it could be effective, agitated as I was. I used a technique performed in the last moments of life, a technique that Joanne, a Healing Touch instructor whom I'd consulted, had kindly taught me. I shook and worked, and Lula watched silently.

Then, up and down, inhale and exhale, Mom's chest began to move. With long, unlabored breaths, she transitioned to a peaceful state, still comatose, but breathing.

Barbara came and went, and Lula went, and a night nursing aide came on. Mom lived for two weeks after that, sometimes awake and relatively alert, but mostly not. Those two hard weeks were perhaps a gift, a moot gift, conferred by a healing art that was neither miracle nor magic.

To Turn or Not To Turn

We had our moments—some really rough ones. Why not? She was dying. And I was no expert at it, this caring for my mother who was lingering so long on no food and teaspoons of liquid that I thought she must be fighting death.

I told her many times it was all right to go. I gave her permission, and over the phone Gail did, too. "You needn't stay for either of us, Mom. We love you, and we'll be fine. So it's okay to go whenever you're ready," I assured her.

I knew how important it was to give such permission—Barbara and Kate had tutored me. Dying people often hang onto life from a sense of duty to their loved ones. They can linger for days past their time until they're given explicit permission to let go.

Despite our assurances, however, Mom hung on, and she grew angry. Then, things got rough. Like the day toward the end when Lula and I prepared to turn her. Standing on either side of her bed, we grasped the draw sheet under her, poised for a pull-and-turn in Lula's direction, in a maneuver that needed repeating every two hours.

"Don't turn me! I want to stay on my back!" Mom commanded.

It had happened the night before, too. I was reading in her room when Mom surfaced into relative consciousness, groaning and holding her right hip.

"Do you want some medicine, Mom?" I asked.

"Leave me alone!" she growled.

"Okay, if that's the way you want it!" I retorted silently.

It wasn't the best way to react, even silently. But at the end of the day at the end of a week at the end of a long, long month, I was frazzled. I got up aggrieved. I grumbled to myself, "I don't want to be sitting in your room, anyway! Let's not pretend it's fun!"

We need to be aware of our anger. We shouldn't deny it or veil it with sugary, strained words. Nor should we yield to it and throw plates or insults. We need to pause and give ourselves space to recognize and investigate what's going on inside.

Investigating anger means noticing where it's located and what it feels like. Is it hot, tight, heavy? Delving into the heart of anger, rather than being caught by the drama that produced it, leads away from it. Facing anger softly, mindfully, is the beginning of freedom from its burden.

Stalking out of Mom's room that evening, I felt my footsteps. They were heavier than usual, and my motions were more angular. I was aware, all right, and there was no softness in it.

"I'll be back soon." I tossed the comment to Maderia, the on-duty nursing aide, as I strode past, making an effort at least to keep the upset from showing in my voice.

I knew it would be wise to meditate in order to become

more centered, but I chose to ignore that option. I gathered my purse and prepared go out to rent a video. "Meditation can wait—losing myself in *Raiders of the Lost Ark* is a good enough way to spend the evening!" I declared truculently. I was silently addressing an invisible spiritual master who seemed to have suddenly established a presence at my shoulder and who was trying to deny me this relaxation. I felt threatened. "I deserve this!" I asserted.

All at once, here was a second anger. On top of my anger at Mom, I'd concocted anger at an imaginary master, whom I was accusing of unfeelingly censuring my actions. It was a big presence to vie with, but I did it, all the way over and back from Blockbuster.

When asked what he was planning to do next, Indiana Jones, in the midst of yet another impossible situation in his quest for the lost ark, replied, "I don't know. I'm makin' this up as I go!"

"Right, Indy. So am I!" I retorted. And as I said it, watching Indiana's acrobatic ride on top of, under, and inside of an enemy's truck, I recognized what was behind my words. Anger doesn't disappear when you avoid it. It transmogrifies and comes back in other contexts, in fiendish little ways.

Indiana's fabulous adventures concluded more or less happily. I achieved a reasonable night's sleep, aided by Sominex, I admit; and in the morning, I meditated. Now, I was standing at Mom's bedside trying to decide, as Indiana had, what to do next.

"Why are you and the nurses doing this to me? Why are you pinning me down?" Mom whined.

I listened aghast. Me—doing this to her?

"Okay, Mom," I conceded. I knew that chemical changes in her brain were probably causing her unreasonableness and that anything I said would make no headway. And I didn't want to use force. I glanced at Lula, signalling to her with my eyes that we should stop our efforts for the moment.

Lula stayed with Mom while I repaired to the kitchen for breakfast and a strategy session. The objective was clear. Regardless of how either of us felt, she had to be turned, because if she remained too long in one position, her skin would break down, and bedsores would develop. Since she hadn't the strength to turn herself, the question was how could we do it without upsetting her.

My last sip of coffee gone, I set down the mug deliberately, watching its white plastic base meet the white, fluted earthenware saucer. The thought floated through my mind that this event had as much validity as any other event in the world at that moment. I wanted to linger with my thoughts and with the mismatched mug and saucer, to examine the shades of whiteness, to explore how their varied glosses kept me at bay on their surface. It wasn't as interesting a study as Indiana and the other raiders, but in this pinch, any distraction would do.

Some awareness pulled me back into the moment, out of the sweet unconscious insulation of reverie. I centered myself and silently declared, "Here goes."

Back in Mom's room, I said quietly, "Mom, we'll let you stay on your back a little while longer, but we'll have to turn you soon."

"Who says?" she demanded.

There was a dragon in that bed! This wasn't the pussy-cat I knew.

"The nurses say. The doctors say." I invoked external authority, knowing my own wouldn't count. I explained about bedsores again. It was an old story to her.

"Who says?" she persisted.

Oh, God!

Then she conceded, "I'm being stubborn, and you are, too."

I agreed. "Yes, we both are."

Worn down by the impasse and by the strain of the days preceding, I searched for an appropriate response, and I found words, not sympathetic ones, but words to the point. It might be the last chance. I, who had so recently been suffering from anger myself, observed, "You've got a choice. You can be angry or else you can accept that your body is dying and let yourself die in peace."

Were they the right words, those hard little stones? Could I take the advice if I were lying in that bed? I don't know. I continued, phrasing my comments in terms I hoped would resonate with her.

"This is God's way. He's calling you like He calls all of us. You're no different, but you have some control here."

Now I was trying to be skillful. Knowing that loss of control was a grief for her, I was trying to identify an area where she still had it, although not the kind she wanted. "You have the control of deciding how you're going to die, angry or not."

"Who says!" A third time.

"Think about it, Mom," I replied, walking out of the room.

Some rough times, yes. Though such acrimony between us was rare, some of the nonacrimonious occasions were no less rough.

About forty-five minutes after I'd left Mom's room, Lula called to me. I was back in my room where I was writing out my pain, covering page after page in my journal with a therapeutic outpouring. Dear journal! It helped me keep some sort of balance during those months of dying and caregiving.

"Your mother wants to talk to you," Lula said.

I didn't rush. I knew Mom had been throwing a temper tantrum. Most of us do when things don't go our way. "The physical world is not answerable to our personal will." The late Reverend Master Jiyu Kennett of Shasta Abbey identified this as one of the laws of the universe. It sounds banal, hardly worth noting, until we encounter the contrariness of life. Then we stamp our feet and jump up and down and scream, "No! I won't accept it!" I speak from personal experience.

A tantrum is a tantrum, regardless of cause, regardless of whether we've been unfairly dealt with or not. The one who suffers most is the thrower, though receivers can be mightily hurt too. Writing about Mom's tantrum made me recognize some of my own, past, as well as my present, blossoming anger at Mom's truculence. It was as if an inner spotlight were shining on some of my dramas. It so sharply illuminated the overall design that it prevented me from submerging, as I often did, in the pain of the details. And it showed me that my refusal to let go of resentment because these events hadn't unfolded my way, in fact, wasn't much different from Mom's reactions now.

I was still thinking about them as I walked slowly to Mom's

room, rephrasing Hamlet's taut query as I went—"To throw or not to throw, that is the question." It was as simple as that. "Yes," or "no." I could let go of my tantrums, or not. Mom could let go of hers and allow herself to be turned, or not.

"Sit down," Mom commanded, motioning for me to sit on the bed next to her.

"I've been sitting. I'll stand," I replied. I wasn't being ornery. I felt that whatever was going to happen, Mom and I needed to meet it on equal ground. Neither of us was in control.

Mom whispered, "We've said some mean things to each other. We never have before. I don't want us to be mean to each other."

Things turned soft inside, and I said, "I don't want to be mean, Mom. I love you. I wish your body were strong and healthy, and I know you do, too. There's nothing we can do about this, but we need to take care of you."

"You don't understand how hard it is for me every time I'm turned—like a mountain is on my body," she explained.

We talked quietly, briefly. Then we struck a deal. She would turn herself if she could, but if not, the nurse and I would help her. And we implemented our deal on the spot.

"Okay, you need to turn on a side." She'd been on her back for almost four hours. Thinking it would be painful for her to lie on her hurting hip, I added, "Why don't you turn away from me?"

"No, I never want to turn away from you."

I leaned down and kissed her, engulfed in a new wave of softness. Straightening, I said, "Hang on. I'll go around to the other side of the bed; then you can turn toward me."

The Twelfth Hour

Alone, my mother had walked into the dim, close room lined with a couple dozen sample coffins, and she chose the one, an amber-colored maple coffin, from which some day she would not arise. It was three years before she died, and at our next Thanksgiving gathering, when the family had assembled from various parts, she informed Gail and Bruce and me what she had done.

Trying to contain emotion behind the fence of her words, and almost succeeding, she explained, "I've made all my funeral arrangements because I don't want you to have to bother when I die. That's no time to be thinking about such business."

It was like her. She didn't want to intrude or burden us. Also, she prized her independence. She wanted as much control as possible over decisions affecting her life and, now, over her death as well.

I appreciated Mom's position, and I admired her courage. Having accompanied her to the mortuary years earlier to arrange for Dad's funeral, I knew that if the paperwork didn't get you, the caskets would. Especially the grim, all-metal number.

Despite Mom's thorough efforts, when her end drew near, final arrangements still remained to be settled. During the last weeks of her life, as she swung between coma and relative responsiveness, I met with the funeral director to review the contract. A graveside funeral, a closed casket, no notice in the newspaper until after the funeral—just as she wanted. Checking each detail, we sat in the same, old-fashioned, leather-chaired office where Mom and I had finalized paperwork for Dad's funeral.

Because the coffin she had selected was no longer available, I needed to make another choice. I entered the casket room whose stillness was like a casket itself. Still, that is, until I arrived, with my surging memories of the occasion when Mom and I had selected Dad's coffin here, and my thoughts of her alone choosing her own, and of all the people who'd ever been in this room in various stages of upset, as I was now. The room wasn't still. It was clamorous with anguish. I picked a casket comparable to the one of Mom's choice, also maple, and I didn't tell her about the change.

My selection made, the director broached the subject of "the death." Almost immediately after the death, he assured me, someone from the mortuary could arrive at our house for the removal of the body.

"Hospice will have to notify us. We can't legally come out before that. But if you call us immediately, we can have a driver ready to leave as soon as we hear from hospice. We'll be out right away to make the removal."

This soft-spoken man was trying so hard to be sensitive and reassuring! He couldn't know that he struck every wrong chord with me. "The death," "the removal"—I needed to discuss this squarely, not in the kid-glove terms in which death is usually addressed in our society. Despite the pioneering work of Elisabeth Kübler-Ross and others after her, despite the growing hospice movement, as a society, we still consider death to be impolite, an embarrassment. In our discomfort and concern lest we distress others and ourselves, we usually avoid the topic or, if that's not possible, we tiptoe around it. This man was tiptoeing.

Beyond the fancy footwork, I was alarmed by the prospect that his words raised—of Mom's body being whisked away before I had a chance to say goodbye. Now you see it; now you don't.

"How much time do I have? Six hours? Twelve?" I blurted. Having been with her day and night for months while she was alive, I suddenly felt I needed to bargain for every minute I could spend with her after she died.

"By law, the remains must be under refrigeration within twenty-four hours of the death," he explained.

"Oh, that's okay," I exhaled in relief. Twenty-four hours was enough time to say goodbye.

"What do you plan to *do* with the body?" he asked, evidently startled that I'd need more time than "right away."

I imagined him conjuring images of my performing bizarre rituals with my mother's body. Defensively, I mumbled a response, but in fact, I had no plans. I didn't know what I would do or how much time would be enough, but I did know I would need to be alone with her. I decided right there on the spot that I wouldn't notify anybody when Mom died, neither hospice nor the mortuary. Not until I was ready.

Collecting myself, I commented, "I gather most people want the body removed right away. Is that right?" I sensed I was bumping into one of our great societal taboos.

"Yes. The family usually has a final viewing, though some are too exhausted to do that. Then we remove the remains."

"The remains"—one moment a person is a living human being and the next, a heap of "remains." Why should he understand my need for more than a "brief viewing"? Why should he understand that one on an inner spiritual path needs to accept death as a natural part of life, a transition to be greeted with the same love and mindfulness with which we try to greet birth and all of the moments in between? We need to live with an awareness of death, not shrink from it.

One morning, a week or so after this meeting, as I walked into her room, Mom commented, "I've been thinking." Early morning was her special thinking time. "I've been thinking about the funeral, and I want to change some things."

"Oh no!" I thought, flinching at the prospect of another meeting at the funeral home.

"I think that a funeral is not something to invite people to." Even in death, she was a private person and didn't want to impose on others.

I was relieved. Another meeting at the mortuary wouldn't be necessary, after all. Then a new concern edged into my mind. This one, I voiced. "But, Mom, a lot of people will want to come to the funeral. You need to remember it's your funeral, but it's theirs, too, in a way. It gives people who love you a chance to say goodbye. They'd be very hurt if they can't come."

Conceding the truth of the point, she stipulated, "Well, okay, but not many, just family and really close friends."

I got pen and paper, and we drew up the list together. I argued, one by one, for the inclusion, beyond the obvious core group, of each person I thought would want to attend. It was almost as though we were in a bazaar haggling over the price of a piece of fabric. We reached a deal, but it was a deal that I must admit I didn't fully honor after her death. There were others who wanted to come, too, and I didn't have the heart to say "no." Gail, who was in town, agreed.

Mom's breath grew loud and labored the afternoon before she died. She lay unresponsive, far away, and phlegm collected in her lungs, making breathing hard. I blamed myself that she was unable to cough it up.

"If only I hadn't given her the Ativan," I chided myself. "Then she'd be more responsive. She'd be able to clear her throat."

My mind jumped with discomfort to an incident a month or so earlier when by mistake, for two and a half days, I'd given Mom Dilaudid. In steady doses, the drug made her retch. I'd thought it was Compazine, a medicine to calm her stomach, because both kinds of suppositories were in the refrigerator. By the third day without improvement, I was exasperated.

"She's convinced herself that she's going to retch, so she's doing it," I thought irritably.

Barbara, who was making one of her biweekly visits as I was preparing to give Mom yet another dose to calm her stomach, looked at the package in my hand and said in a low, hushed voice, "That's Dilaudid, not Compazine."

Oh, God! I debated whether to tell Mom and apologize, but I decided not to. It would serve no good purpose to shake her faith in me as the keeper and dispenser of her medicine.

Now, a month later, I was agonizing over whether I'd botched it again. As on so many other occasions, I called hospice. The nurse on phone duty assured me that my mother's wheezing had nothing to do with medication. This was terminal congestion, the death rattle.

I'd heard about the death rattle many times in novels and on television. Barbara had carefully described it. Now I listened to it first-hand. I listened to the prelude to the final stage for which Mom had been waiting for weeks.

All that day and that night, almost without thought, I listened. And I meditated and co-meditated with her, trying to match the pace of my breathing to hers, but, most of all, I just sat numbly. And that night I lay numbly on sofa cushions on the floor in her room, still listening to each breath—in and out—listening as, in the early morning, her breathing underwent subtle changes, growing lighter but not easy. Finally, a little before 6:00 a.m., her breath grew very light.

When there could be no doubt regarding what was about to happen, I asked the nursing aide to leave. Yvonne had spent the night in a chair at the kitchen table. I was glad she was there, though neither of us could do much for Mom. Walking Yvonne to the door on that still cool, sunny July morning, I saw a single deer, grazing on the lawn. It raised its head, and we looked at each other for a long moment. I went back to the bed where

Mom lay unconscious, and I told her. She would have liked that deer. Then, I listened again, standing by her bed. I watched her draw each light breath, until she did not take another.

Over the years, I'd studied various religions' views on death, but I learned something new that morning. I learned that bodily death doesn't happen when we stop breathing. It happens gradually. Holding Mom's hands and kissing her forehead during the next hour or so after her last breath, I felt them slowly grow cold, as did her feet. But even more than an hour later, the back of her neck and torso were still warm. Those cells, near her heart, had not yet died.

I needed to touch Mom's body, to kiss her, just as I needed to cry and to meditate and pray next to her. It was part of my goodbye. Touching her was also part of my way of facing mortality. I had wanted to walk with Mom as far as is possible for a person to accompany another to the realm of death. And I was doing it. And now that death was here, I wanted to be close as she underwent it.

Although I let my actions unfold without an agenda during the hours following her death, I knew clearly what I would *not* do. I would not do anything that she would have been uncomfortable with in life. No candles. No Buddhist scriptures. In fact, no scriptures at all. Although deeply rooted in Judaism, Mom seldom turned to the Bible. Bible stories weren't part of her conversation. Once, during her final illness, thinking she might have grown more receptive, I read some Psalms to her. She listened politely, without comment. When I offered to read more the next day, she waved her hand and said, "Read something else."

I left the Bible by her bed, though—just in case.

Amid the solemnity of the last morning, as I sat next to Mom's body, my stomach rumbled. Irreverently, it reminded me that it was breakfast time. Life can be so inappropriate!

"This is awkward—Mom has just died, and you're hungry!" I admonished my stomach. Actually, I appreciated my stomach's sense of humor.

I brought breakfast into her room, because next to her was the only place I wanted to be. "You know, Mom," I said, sitting at her bedside munching cereal, "some people might think this is a little morbid."

I could almost hear her laugh.

About two hours later, as Gail was waking up in Los Angeles, I called her. The news was no surprise since we'd been talking regularly. Knowing Mom's time was near, she was preparing to come to St. Louis for the funeral. Then I called hospice. (Later, I learned that hospice people had been surprised I'd waited so long to inform them. I had guarded my intentions well.) I requested that the hearse from the mortuary not be sent for another hour and a half. Though I was ready to make the hospice call, I wasn't ready yet to part with Mom.

Meanwhile, my cousin Sherry, who had been out of town on business, returned early, knowing intuitively what had happened. She arrived at the house in time to watch the hearse slowly pull out of the driveway.

The tehara was my last chance to be with Mom before the funeral. A beautiful Jewish ritual involving washing the body of the deceased before burial, the tehara is performed as a service by a society whose volunteers are trained in the complex rite.

When I'd settled the final funeral arrangements a few weeks earlier, the funeral director had asked if we wanted a tehara. "It's optional, and your mother wasn't clear about it," he explained, informing me of the added cost.

"We want it if I can take part," I responded immediately. Then inwardly sorting through reasons to justify my unilateral decision, I located some good ones. Mom had talked about ritual washings in recent months, and I knew she wasn't opposed. Additionally, it was better to conclude the matter at this meeting, rather than trying to find an appropriate time to discuss it with Mom and having to come back to the funeral home later to sign the final contract. It made sense, but the truth was that I deeply wanted to participate in the ceremony. The tehara was as much for me as for her.

He hesitated. "Jewish law prohibits children from viewing their parents' naked bodies."

Gripped by my wish to participate, I dismissed a few thousand years of Jewish law without a qualm. "I've been tending to my mother's intimate functions for months, so that hardly seems relevant," I observed dryly.

He agreed to try to work it out. At the time, I assumed that this was one of those laws that sometimes is honored in the breach, that occasionally other determined offspring had participated in their parent's tehara. Later, however, the funeral director told me that this was the first instance he had encountered in his years in the profession. "I agreed to see if it could be done because I wanted to be of service," he explained.

Later, it occurred to me that there may be another reason for the prohibition, more practical than Jewish law: a weepy, squeamish daughter would be a problem at her mother's tehara. I had no guarantee that I wouldn't be weepy and squeamish.

Apparently others weren't sure, either. Or maybe their reservations were strictly legal. In any case, prior to the tehara, I received two or three calls from people connected with the event, each voicing hesitation, as though testing my resolve.

When the time came, I was, in fact, neither weepy nor squeamish. The tehara was performed at the mortuary early in the morning on the day of the funeral. Having received permission to participate, reluctant though it had been, I was now fully welcomed into the ritual. In a precise, unsentimental way, the four women volunteers, none of whom knew my mother, explained each step as they performed it, and they quietly showed me how to join in.

One woman, who was reciting Hebrew prayers over Mom's body, turned to me and offered a sheet of paper covered with Hebrew script. "Would you like to recite the prayers?" she asked softly.

"I can't read Hebrew, thank you," I demurred.

At that moment, I realized this was an unusual situation indeed. "These women probably think I'm a lapsed Jew. They don't know how lapsed," I thought. "A Buddhist participating in her mother's tehara can't be an everyday event."

At the end of the proceedings, with my mother's body cleaned, dressed in simple white burial garments, and closed in the satin-lined, maple coffin, I thanked each of the women.

I looked into their eyes, and I saw strength—four women doing what needed to be done, with reverence, a sacred act performed without hesitation or false piety, no flippancy borne of fear. What a relief! What a fitting preparation for my strong mother, who later that day went to her grave, next to her beloved Stoney, in the presence, as she had wished, of her two daughters, her son-in-law, and a small group of family and friends.

Here

Medford and points north. Standing in the Greyhound terminal in Redding, California, waiting to board the northbound bus for Mt. Shasta, I am on my way back. Two months after Mom's death, I am going back to the Abbey for the first time in over a year. A short visit, this, but a needed retreat.

"Big bag checked at the baggage counter, small zippered bag on the floor by my feet, purse on my shoulder with ticket—everything accounted for." My mental survey completed, I idly regard the bank of closed glass doors in front of me, four leading out and one for coming in. With different destinations marked above each, the doors give onto the same traffic. I spot a metaphor. Lives go in diverse directions, but we're all trafficking in the same basic issues. "Can I get to Medford if I walk through the Sacramento door? Intending one place, don't we often end up some place else? I have."

Gazing at the busyness beyond, I wonder how I've changed since I last stood here at the end of Mom's chemotherapy many months ago, waiting to walk through the Medford door. I wonder, but only for a moment, because the answer, whatever it is, doesn't seem to matter. "I've changed as I've changed. That's enough to know."

Into the waiting space that stretches around me, into the dawdling minutes, my attention wanders. To a square, sixty-ish woman in front of me in line—to her permed purple-gray hair, navy polyester slacks, gum-soled shoes and her capacious purse for traveling. "Not much older than I am," I admit to myself reluctantly, wanting to turn away. "Age is just age" is still a hard one for me. She is going to Tacoma to visit her sister and brother-in-law. I learn that and more later, when, with a fresh mindset, I sit next to her on the bus.

In front of her in line is a young couple, quietly absorbed in each other's presence. You can tell they're close because they dress like twins, all in black—pants, shirts, sneakers—she with a gold nose ring, he with a matching ring in his ear. Inspecting her and her spiky hair, I wonder if her nose is really pierced or if the ring is fake, the kind they sell to scare your mother.

"Probably real," I conclude. "She doesn't look like the type who cares if she scares her mother or not." I am laying on judgements like I spread peanut butter on bread. "And he—" I turn a critical mind to him, ready with another dollop.

Such judgements are unkind, of course. More than that, they're sneaky. They creep around, waiting for a chance to catch you unaware and, finding it, they lock you in the hothouse of your mind where you can turn rancid without even noticing. My spiritual training usually alerts me to their presence. Now, however, submerged in boredom, I'm a prime target. Judgements are poised for a high time with me until, suddenly, a young mother barges through the in-door, close after her son.

"Stay with me, Billy! Hold my hand!" she scolds. And, all unwittingly, she jolts me out of my torpor.

She doesn't wait for Billy to respond, clearly sensing a lost cause. She lunges for his hand, but he, pulling down with shoulder and arm, wiggles free and bolts. Head down, dodging adults, his small, yellow tee-shirted figure flees into the lobby. His mother pursues, yelling. I watch. No one else seems to pay much attention, least of all Billy, whose actions suggest a future of maternal grief. Or is his a fleeting petulance, the unleashing of young-boy energies too long confined to the bus?

Leaving mother and son to work out their differences in the lobby, I sigh, "I've seen this before." Wearily I begin to slip back into comparison. "Well, not *this* exactly, but other mothers here tending children with uneven success."

Here. My attention shifts carelessly, critically to the place: a worn building in the midst of a tired downtown in a featureless city at the tip-end of California's central valley—a little remote, a little dreary. Another spot on the way to somewhere else. Another step.

My flittering thoughts begin to launch into a review of selected events in my life that bring me finally to this place. I know what's coming—it's a well-trod route, this review of events, especially recent, painful ones, to which my emotions still flock in bunches. They're like pigeons in their winter roosting place—flock and fly, flock and fly.

As the review gets under way, the phrase from the Lotus Ceremony that I've heard many times before sounds in my mind. I hear it softly, as background music to the dramas at hand—"wandering in training one step at a time."

In St. Louis, I focused on the step-by-step meaning in the phrase. It was a guidepost of sorts. "Yes," I think, shifting my weight from one foot to the other, "I've been doing that—"

All at once I know—really know, not just think—that "wandering" doesn't mean "lost." It doesn't mean "on the road to somewhere else." All at once, I know that this "wandering" is deeper. It means living unconditionally, letting go into right here, into the unique texture of this moment, each moment.

Hereness—open-ended and utterly focused at the same time. Its very lack of structure forms a bright scaffold, an unseen support that I suddenly perceive more strongly than I perceive my own body. Astonishing! Because there is no need to grab the handrail of my opinions or check the solidity of the flooring of my beliefs. They are insignificant and always will be. The inner structure of the moment supports me, whether I feel lost or not. "I'm on my way to the Abbey, yes, but what I'm looking for there is right here, too, in the Greyhound terminal. The question is whether I access it, and how deeply."

I relax into this hereness, which is blooming as an intense and sacred presence in my body. I relax into the wonderful bazaar of noise and smells and colors around me, into the tension between Billy and his frazzled mother, into the passion of the twins, into an awareness that the gray-haired woman in front is more than simply a mirror for my struggle with aging. I laugh. The space, the fun of it!

I relax too into knowing that this sense of hereness will grow dull, then fade away. As it has before, in St. Louis and elsewhere. But it will be back, maybe more often now. Or maybe not. Either way, there is only offering, offering. . . .